JANE'S 1982-83 AVIATION REVIEW

JANE'S 1982-83
AVIATION REVIEW

edited by Michael J.H. Taylor

Second year of issue

JANE'S

Copyright © Jane's Publishing Company Limited 1982

First published in 1982 by
Jane's Publishing Company Limited
238 City Road, London EC1V 2PU

Distributed in Canada, the Philippines and the USA and
its dependencies by
Science Books International Inc
51 Sleeper Street, Boston, MA 02210

ISBN 0 86720 632 2

Designed by Bernard Crossland Associates

Printed in the United Kingdom by
Netherwood Dalton & Co Ltd
Huddersfield

Publisher's note
The first compilation in this series, published in October
1981, was issued under the title *Jane's Aviation Annual
1981-82*.

Contents

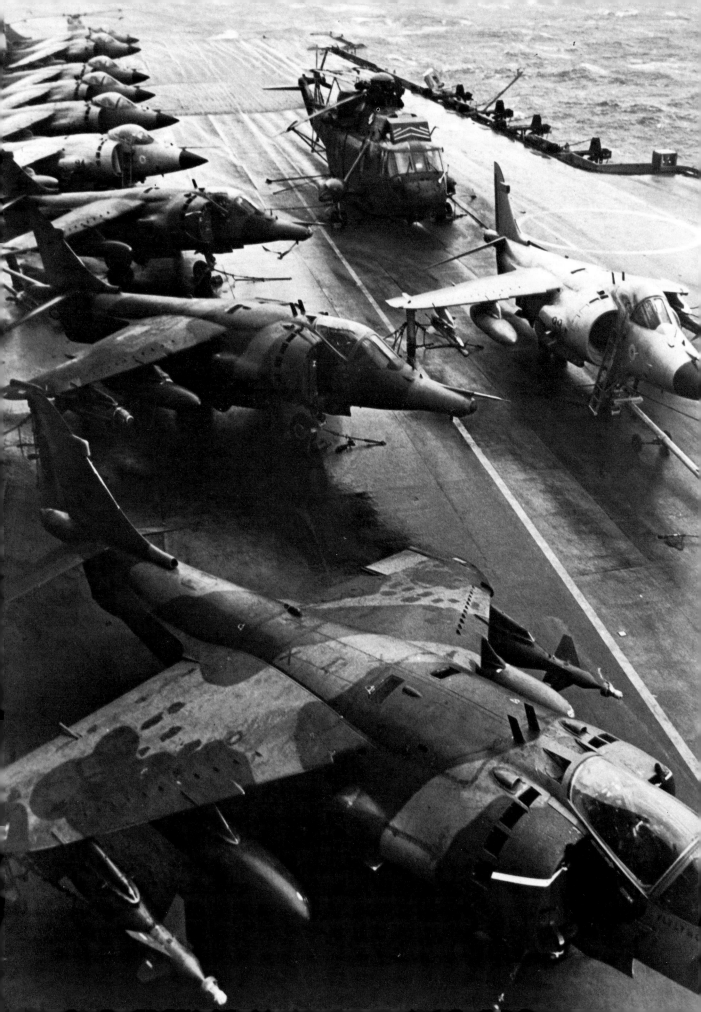

Introduction

The day this introduction was written, news came through from the Falkland Islands that the fighting there had stopped. This conflict gave rise to many questions, the single most important of which was how two friendly nations could find themselves at war. Several of these questions are discussed in the first article of this year's *Jane's Aviation Review, Wings for the Third World*, and there is no need to add more here. However, nobody could fail to be impressed by the courage and tenacity of the pilots on both sides. Whatever the political repercussions, the qualities of the pilots proved to be of the very highest order.

But what of the Sea Harrier? Is it really as good a fighting aircraft as initial reports indicated? Some years ago Harriers were matched in mock combat against four US fighters, which included the USAF's McDonnell Douglas F-15 Eagle and the Navy's Grumman F-14 Tomcat. The outcome was staggering. On average four out of every five combats that ended with a decisive winner went to the Harrier. Little wonder that the USMC, as much as the British services, has been responsible for the impetus behind the continuing development of Harrier into the AV-8B Harrier II. Inevitably some fundamentalists thought the Harrier too slow and too lightly armed with missiles to replace the more conventional naval fighters. Increasing further the Harrier's air-to-air armament could be worthwhile but, as the Battle of Britain showed four decades ago, close air battles are rarely fought at the highest speeds. A more important question must be whether Britain's *Invincible*-class carriers, lacking provision for on-board airborne early-warning aircraft when *Invincible* went to war in the South Atlantic and now carrying hurriedly converted AEW Sea Kings, are themselves adequately protected and capable of providing realistic air cover for other vessels.

It is unrealistic to rely totally and in the long term on AEW cover from Sea Kings or the RAF's new Nimrod AEW3. Apart from the obvious operating limitations, a number of experts doubt the survivability of conventional Awacs aircraft under war conditions. The answer could be the use of easily stowable RPVs, launched from carrier decks to remain airborne for long periods. Such vehicles would have other advantages, although the concept would undoubtedly be very hard to sell. These aircraft could be virtually undetectable to an enemy, whose first concern in war would be to eliminate airborne eyes. An extremely small radar signature and the ability to operate at very high altitudes make this option highly attractive.

On another military front, visitors to Farnborough 82 were able to see for the first time outside the USA the awesome Rockwell International B-1. One hundred of these bombers are destined for service with the USAF in the second half of this decade. However, it is sobering to remember that while the B-1 programme has been cut, restarted and reduced in numbers to save money, the Soviet Union has not only steadily increased the number of its supersonic Backfire bombers but is flight-testing an even more formidable supersonic bomber known to NATO as Blackjack.

On the commercial front, Concorde's future remains in doubt as the money-men decide whether it would be cheaper to scrap the world's most advanced airliner or keep it flying. Whatever the outcome, Concorde has proved reliable, utterly safe and extremely popular, and has given the British and French aircraft industries experience in design and construction that is unique. Concorde also had a part to play during the first days of the Falklands crisis, carrying British politicians speedily to the United States. It cannot be argued that Concorde should be operated purely as a time-saving trans-

The crowded flight deck of Task Force flagship HMS *Hermes* on a stormy day during the Falklands war. Visible are three RAF Harrier GR3s — the one in the foreground is armed with Paveway laser-guided bombs — seven Royal Navy Sea Harrier FRS1s and a Sea King anti-submarine helicopter. *(MoD)*

Front cover **Falklands figurehead: Sea Harrier chocked and chained on the ski-jump ramp of HMS** *Hermes. (Press Association)*

atlantic airbridge for politicians, although one such aircraft for use by the Cabinet and Royal Family could make sense. But the political effects of a journey by the Foreign Secretary to the US in the shortest possible time are paralleled in the world of commerce. Who can judge how many millions of pounds have been earned by the speed at which executives have seized transatlantic opportunities? Viability should be judged on more than the bald equation of fuel, maintenance and operating costs versus direct revenue.

This year's *Jane's Aviation Review* provides an insight into the latest aerospace technologies, discusses the Laker collapse and the latest innovations from American Burt Rutan, that master of uniquely configured aeroplanes, and describes the massive aviation effort in the Bright Star joint military manoeuvres in Egypt. For followers of lighter-than-air and rotor-craft, there are articles on the future of cargo-carrying airships and the incredible world of the Wallis autogyros. Containing contributions from some of the world's most respected aerospace writers, the *Review* offers a panoramic view of the aviation world of today and tomorrow, while yesterday gets its due in *Jarrett's Jubilees*.

MJHT

Publisher's note The word "Annual" has been replaced with "Review" in the title of this book and its military and naval companions to avoid any possible confusion with our yearbooks amongst booksellers. The edition date has been dropped from the cover for the same reason.

The Contributors

Peter W. Brooks took an honours degree in engineering and learned to fly before beginning his career as an aviation journalist. After a period as air correspondent of an evening paper he served in the Second World War as an operational pilot on aircraft carriers and as a naval test pilot. After the war he became a technical officer at the Ministry of Civil Aviation and then, for ten years, worked for British European Airways. Between then and his present appointment as regional executive for Europe in the Aircraft Group headquarters of British Aerospace he spent a number of years as joint managing director of Beagle Aircraft Ltd and as manager (international collaboration) with BAC.

Susan J. Bushell is the youngest contributor to the *Aviation Review*. She is joint compiler of *Airshows*, an annual publication listing all aircraft participating at air events throughout the calendar year. She works as an editorial assistant and writer with *Aviation News*, and is also an aviation photographer and picture researcher.

Don Downie is an aviation reporter and photographer. He is a member of the Aviation/Space Writers Association and the Society of Experimental Test Pilots. During the Second World War he became a flight instructor and transport pilot in India, being awarded the Air Medal with cluster and DFC with cluster. As a post-war commercial pilot he logged more than 10,000 hours in the air. Author of ten books on aviation and more than 1,000 magazine articles, he still enjoys flying as a member of AOPA and EAA and owns a 1952 Cessna 170B.

Terry Gander spent five years in the RAF, specialising in air radar. After leaving the service he went into the new and expanding technology of computers, joining Rank Xerox. Some years later he began writing on military subjects, specialising in artillery and other weapons systems, and is currently on the staff of *Jane's Defence Review*.

Alan W. Hall was trained as a graphic artist and taught in schools of art at Malvern and Stafford before going to the London School of Printing in 1956. He was then studio manager of a firm of industrial publishers, and later art director of a West End advertising agency.

Founder editor of *Airfix Magazine* in 1960. Public relations officer at successively, the Ministry of Aviation, Heathrow Airport and, for eight years, RAE Farnborough. Started *Aviation News* as publisher/editor in 1972, took complete control of the business in 1974 and started *Scale Aircraft Modelling* in 1978.

Philip Jarrett AMRAeS has been writing on aviation history since 1967. After eight years at the Royal Aeronautical Society, first as library assistant and then as assistant editor on the newspaper *Aerospace*, he became assistant editor of *Aeroplane Monthly* when that journal was launched in 1973. He is now production editor of *Flight International*. Specialising in early aviation history, he has contributed papers and articles to a variety of aviation publications.

Roy McLeavy is an acknowledged expert on hovercraft and other surface-skimming vehicles, and has written widely on the subject. He has been the editor of *Jane's Surface Skimmers* since it was first published 15 years ago.

David Mondey FRHistS, AMRAeS, formerly an engineer in the Royal Air Force, has become well known internationally as an aviation author. He has written or edited more than 20 aviation books, the most recent including *Planemakers 2: Westland* and *Giants in the Sky*, and compiles the US aircraft section of *Jane's All the World's Aircraft*.

Kenneth Munson AMRAeS, ARHistS has contributed to *Jane's All the World's Aircraft* since 1968, becoming assistant editor with special responsibility for much of the main aircraft section, sailplanes, microlights and hang-gliders in 1973. He has produced more than 40 books, the latest being *US Commercial Aircraft* (Jane's), a picture portfolio depicting the great types in American airline history.

Michael J. H. Taylor is a full-time aviation author and editor with more than 35 books to his credit over the past 13 years. His most recent publications include *Fantastic Flying Machines* and *Planemakers 1: Boeing*. He compiles the homebuilt aircraft section of *Jane's All the World's Aircraft* and is the editor of and major contributor to the five-volume *Jane's Encyclopedia of Aviation*.

John W. R. Taylor FRAeS, FRHistS, FSLAET began his aviation career in 1941 as a member of Sir Sydney Camm's wartime fighter design team at Hawker Aircraft Ltd. He has led for 22 years the team responsible for *Jane's All the World's Aircraft*, the bible of the aerospace industry. The 215 books bearing his name, published in more than twelve languages, include everything from spotters' handbooks to an award-winning history of the RAF Central Flying School and a history of aviation of which more than 280,000 copies have been sold worldwide.

William H. Turner V soloed on a Curtiss OX-5 Robin when he was just twelve years old, later becoming a pilot with the US Navy and thereafter a law school dean. Following an early retirement at 50, he began the construction of replica racing aircraft and currently owns and flies the replica 1931 Gee Bee *City of Springfield* and 1934 Brown Racer *Miss Los Angeles*. Under construction in 1982 is a replica of the British de Havilland D.H.88 Comet, the twin-engined racer built originally to compete in the MacRobertson England-Australia Air Race.

Reginald Turnill, internationally known aerospace writer and broadcaster, was the BBC's aerospace correspondent from 1958 to 1976. He began his writing and reporting career during the 1930s, covering many of the most important aviation events of the period. The launch of Sputnik 1 in 1957 prompted his specialisation in spaceflight, and at present he is space editor of BBC's *Newsround* and editor of and principal contributor to *Jane's Spaceflight Directory*.

Wing Commander Kenneth Horatio Wallis CEng, FRAeS, FRSA is one of the most respected names in aviation today, having contributed greatly to the advancement of autogyro design and application. He was introduced to aviation at an early age by his father and uncle, who had designed and built what was probably the first aeroplane to employ steel tubing for its primary structure, the Wallbro monoplane of 1910. He became an amateur constructor of high-speed watercraft in the early 1930s and gained his pilot's licence in April 1937. First joining the Civil Air Guard and then the RAFVR, he was commissioned in the RAF in 1940. After a period flying Westland Lysander army co-operation aircraft he converted to Vickers Wellington bombers and flew 36 missions over Germany and Italy, instructing between operational tours. His first homebuilt ultra-light autogyro flew in 1961, and three years later he left the RAF as a qualified jet pilot to form Wallis Autogyros Ltd. During 1968-9 his autogyros took the first of many world records for altitude and speed in their class. Since then he has used his aircraft in collaboration with aerospace companies, the Home Office and scientific establishments, and the film industry.

Chronology

June 1, 1981—June 22, 1982

DAVID MONDEY

1981

June 1
First flight of G-ROOM, prototype of the Shorts 360 36-seat twin-turboprop commuter transport.

June 4
The Swiss Government announced approval of the purchase for the Swiss Air Force of 40 Pilatus PC-7/CH Turbo Trainers, with deliveries to begin in October 1982.

June 5
Flying a specially prepared Rutan Long-EZ lightplane, Richard G. Rutan set a world straight-line distance record in FAI Class C-1-b of 7,344.56km (4,563.7 miles).

June 6
Air France announced its order for 25 Airbus Industrie A320s, with options on an additional 25.

June 7
Eight Israeli Air Force F-16s, escorted by F-15s, attacked the Osirak nuclear reactor near Baghdad, Iraq, prompting the United States to impose a temporary embargo on the supply of further F-16s to Israel.

June 15
Mr Agha Shahi, the Pakistan Foreign Minister, stated in Islamabad that the United States had agreed to supply General Dynamics F-16s to the Pakistan Air Force.

June 16
The first Sikorsky CH-53E Super Stallion assault transport helicopter for service with the US Marine Corps was handed over officially at Stratford, Connecticut.

June 17
The third prototype of the Panavia Tornado F2 (A.03) was flown for the first time with the new Foxhunter air interception radar developed by Marconi Avionics.

June 19
The Boeing Vertol Model 234 Commercial Chinook 44-seat transport helicopter gained FAA certification. British certification by the CAA followed later in the month.

Rutan Long-EZ flown by Richard "Dick" Rutan. *(Downie and Associates)*

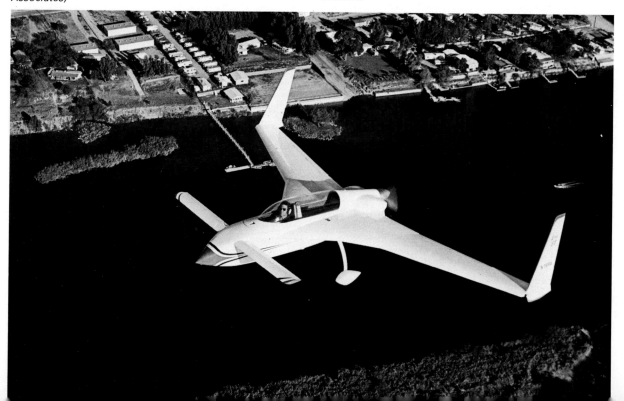

June 25

The UK Defence Secretary announced that the government intended to procure 60 McDonnell Douglas AV-8Bs for service with the RAF under the designation Harrier GR5.

June 26

Pan American highlighted the serious financial problems facing the world's airlines by selling eight of its Boeing 747s to a credit corporation. The resulting cash infusion eased the airline's problems and it is now leasing back the same eight aircraft.

June 26

The first production Grumman/General Dynamics EF-111A (66-049) made its first flight. This is a specially developed tactical jamming aircraft for service with the US Air Force.

June 30

Eastern Airways, of Humberside Airport, Kirmington, Lincolnshire, took delivery of its first Shorts 330, to be used on the company's commuter routes within the UK.

July 1

The first Grumman G-111, a commuter conversion of the HU-16 Albatross military amphibian, entered service with Chalks International Airline on the route between Fort Lauderdale, Florida, and Paradise Island, Nassau. The conversion from military to civil configuration was carried out by Grumman.

Grumman G-111 flown by Chalks International Airline.

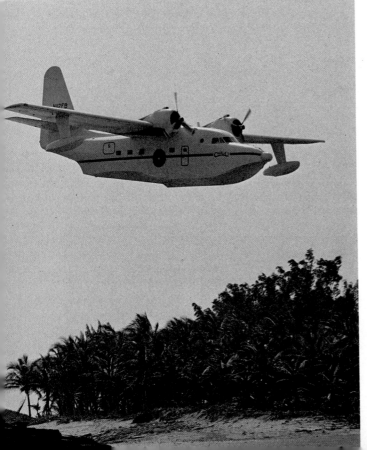

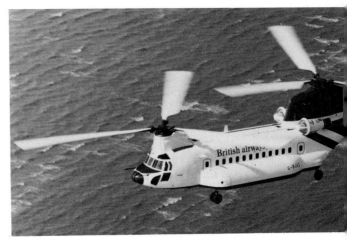

British Airways Helicopters Boeing Model 234.

July 1

British Airways Helicopters introduced the first of its Boeing Model 234s into commercial service, operating the aircraft on contract flights to North Sea gas/oil platforms.

July 2

The Swiss Government signed a letter of agreement with Northrop covering the supply of an additional 32 F-5E and six two-seat F-5F combat aircraft for the Swiss Air Force. Terms of the agreement include manufacture and sub-assembly of various components at Emmen, plus final assembly.

July 3

Aeroflot inaugurated its first international service with the Ilyushin Il-86 wide-body transport, operating the type on the Moscow-East Berlin route.

July 7

The MacCready Solar Challenger made the first crossing of the English Channel by a solar-powered aircraft. Pilot for the 5hr 23min, 156 nm (290km; 180 miles) flight from Cergy-Pontoise, near Paris, to Manston Airfield, Kent, was Steve Ptacek.

July 8

A reconstructed airfield was opened at Glenrothes New Town, Scotland, as Fife Airport. The new airport has a 700m (2,300ft) hard runway which was built with financial aid from the European Regional Development Fund.

July 14

A Grumman F-14 Tomcat made the type's first flight under the power of two General Electric F101-DFE (Definitive Fighter Engine) advanced augmented turbofans.

July 15

The first Lockheed TR-1A single-seat tactical reconnaissance aircraft for service with the US Air Force was rolled out at Palmdale, California.

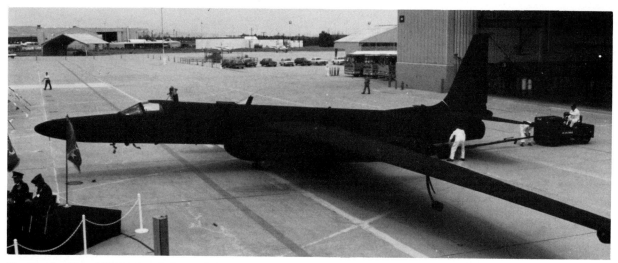

The first Lockheed TR-1A is rolled out. *(USAF)*

July 17
First flight of the prototype of the Piper T-1040, a turboprop-powered commuter airliner developed from the PA-31-350 Chieftain. It is to be marketed by a new organisation, the Airline Division, which Piper established on June 4, 1981.

July 23
A new altitude record for helicopters in FAI Class E-1-d was set by Charles Praether in an Agusta A.109A at Philadelphia, Pennsylvania. The record has since been ratified by the FAI at a height of 6,096m (20,000ft). Two time-to-height records were set at the same time.

July 30
Beech Aircraft began deliveries of the 15-passenger Commuter C99 airliner following the receipt of FAA certification.

July 31
The Japan Maritime Self-Defence Agency signed a contract with Grumman for the supply of four additional E-2C Hawkeye AEW aircraft; two were scheduled for delivery in 1984 and two in 1985.

July 31
Flight trials of Ferranti's new FIN 1064 inertial navigation system aboard a Sepecat Jaguar began at Warton, Lancashire. Apart from having much increased computer capacity, the FIN 1064 is some 50kg (110lb) lighter and one third of the volume of the INS it replaces.

August 1
Japan Air Lines celebrated the 30th anniversary of its foundation as a civil airline.

August 1
The first section of Saab-Scania's new factory at Linkoping, built for production of the Saab-Fairchild 340, was handed over by the contractor.

August 1
First flight of the first Lockheed TR-1A tactical reconnaissance aircraft (80-1066) at Palmdale, California.

August 3
Boeing attained a new production milestone with the delivery of its 4,000th jetliner, a 727-200 for Ansett Airlines of Australia.

Boeing Model 727-200 in Ansett Airlines of Australia livery. *(Boeing)*

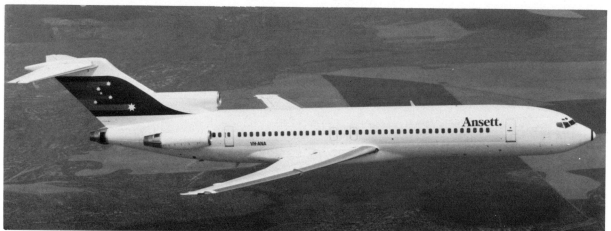

August 4

The first Boeing 767 prototype (N767BA) was rolled out at Everett, Washington.

August 8

The F-16 Fighting Falcon was grounded following a fatal accident. On completion of remedial modifications the aircraft were cleared for operational use on August 18.

August 14

The second Boeing E-3A Sentry Awacs aircraft for service with Nato was delivered to Dornier at Oberpfaffenhofen for installation of its AEW avionics.

August 14

A Defence White Paper prepared by the Japanese Defence Agency claimed that the Soviet Union was deploying 2,210 tactical aircraft in the Far East. The total included some 1,600 fighters and fighter-bombers.

August 15

The McDonnell Douglas DC-8-71, a DC-8 Super Sixty fitted with CFM56 turbofans, made a successful 5hr first flight.

August 18

The Portuguese Air Force received the first of 20 Vought A-7P Corsair IIs. These are refurbished A-7As with avionics to A-7E standard.

August 24

Canadair announced that development of the stretched CL-610 Challenger E business/commuter transport had been postponed indefinitely.

August 26

First flight of the first McDonnell Douglas F-15J Eagle to be assembled by Mitsubishi in Japan from US-built components.

McDonnell Douglas DC-10 with winglets.

August 28

The US Defense Department announced that McDonnell Douglas had been selected as prime contractor for development of the proposed CX transport aircraft.

August 31

The Thai Government announced that 20 N22B Nomad multi-role aircraft had been ordered for service with the Royal Thai Air Force. Government Aircraft Factories in Australia was scheduled to begin deliveries during 1982.

August 31

A McDonnell Douglas DC-10 made a first flight with drag-reducing winglets installed at the wingtips. It marked the beginning of a flight test programme to evaluate the effect of the winglets on fuel economy.

September 3

McDonnell Douglas delivered its 1,000th DC-9, a Super 80 (HB-INO) for service with Swissair.

September 3

G-SSSH, prototype of the British Aerospace 146 Series 100 four-turbofan short-range transport, made a successful first flight at Hatfield, Hertfordshire.

September 7

Edwin A. Link, inventor of the Link Trainer, died at the age of 77. His ground-based trainer was the first stepping-stone towards the sophisticated simulators now used for a major portion of all flight training.

September 10

First flight, at Mojave, California, of the Fairchild/Ames 62 per cent scale example of the NGT (Next Generation Trainer) T-37 replacement which Fairchild has submitted to the US Air Force.

September 11

Bell Helicopter announced development of the Ring Fin helicopter anti-torque device. It comprises a flat ring located near the plane of a small-diameter tail

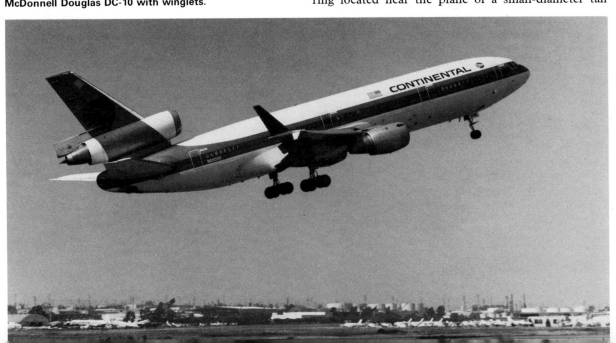

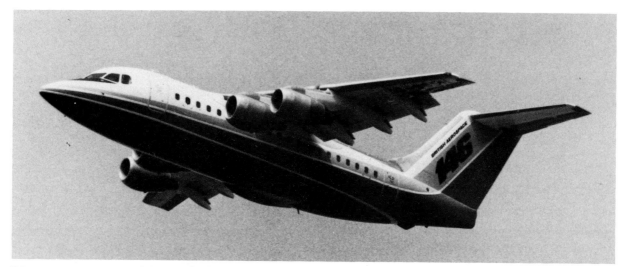

BAe 146 Series 100 prototype G-SSSH. (BAe)

Bell Ring Fin helicopter anti-torque device. (Bell)

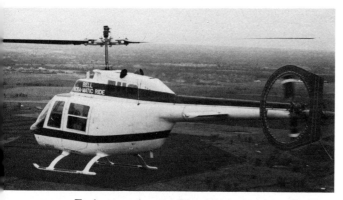

rotor. Early tests showed Ring Fin to be very effective, and an extended trials programme was projected.

September 13
The 50th anniversary of the flight by Flt Lt John Boothman RAF in a Supermarine S.6B high-speed seaplane which won the Schneider Trophy outright for the UK.

September 15
The 494th Tactical Fighter Squadron, based at RAF Lakenheath, Suffolk, became the first US Air Force unit to be declared operational with the Pave Tack weapon-delivery system. The Pave Tack pod houses a laser transmitter/receiver and a precision optical sight.

September 17
Following evaluation of the F-5S version of the Tiger-shark, F-16 Fighting Falcon, F-18 Hornet and the Mirage 2000, the Saab 2105 was recommended as the most suitable aircraft to meet the Swedish Air Force's JAS multi-role fighter requirement.

September 20
First flight of a Sepecat Jaguar fitted with a Marconi Avionics/Dowty quadruplex electrically signalled flight control system with no mechanical backup.

Sepecat Jaguar with fly-by-wire control system. (BAe)

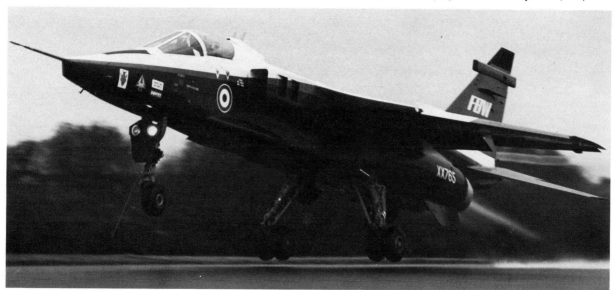

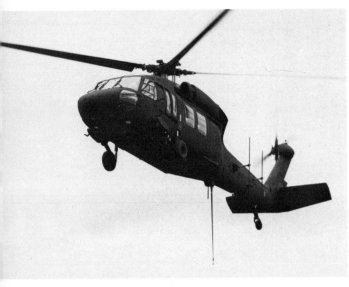

Sikorsky YEH-60A prototype. *(Sikorsky)*

September 20
The People's Republic of China launched three satellites into Earth orbit with a single booster. It was the nation's first multiple launch.

September 20
A new UK operator, Anglo-Scottish Air Parcels, began a twice-daily small parcel delivery service between nine UK airports.

September 21
It was announced that Bell Helicopter had won the US Army's Armed Helicopter Improvement Program (AHIP) contest. An initial $148 million contract was to be awarded to cover the design, modification and test of five prototypes. Bell could receive an estimated $1,000 million contract to modify 720 OH-58A Kiowas to AHIP configuration.

First flight of the Boeing Model 767.

September 22
An Ilyushin Il-86 captained by G. Volokhov established for the Soviet Union a new world speed record in its class, carrying payloads of 35,000-65,000kg at a speed of 526.3kt (975.3km/hr, 606.02mph) over a 2,000km closed circuit. Two days later the same aircraft/pilot combination set a new record over a 1,000km closed circuit of 519.1kt (962km/hr, 597.8mph) with payloads of 30,000-80,000kg.

September 24
First flight of the prototype Sikorsky EH-60A communications-jamming version of the UH-60 Black Hawk helicopter.

September 25
The first production Panavia Tornado for the Italian Air Force, dual-control trainer IT.001, made its first flight at Caselle. It was scheduled for delivery to the Trinational Tornado Training Establishment at RAF Cottesmore in early 1982.

September 25
The 11-seat Piper T-1020 commuter airliner made its first flight.

September 26
First flight of the Boeing 767, from Paine Field, Everett, Washington State. The 2hr 4min flight was made three days ahead of a target set in 1978.

September 28
The Skyship 500 non-rigid airship (G-BIHN), built by Airship Industries (formerly Aerospace Developments), made a successful two-hour first flight at RAF Cardington, Bedfordshire.

September 30
The last de Havilland Comet airline flight in the UK, by Comet 4C G-BOIX from Lasham, Hampshire, to the Royal Scottish Museum site at East Fortune.

October 2
President Reagan announced that 100 Rockwell B-1B

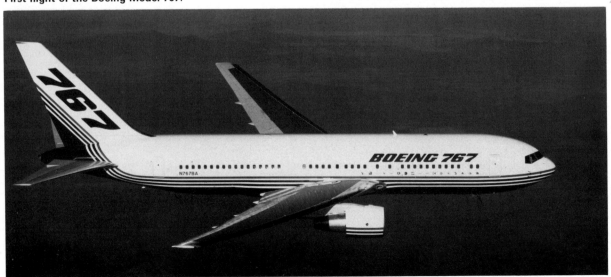

SAL (Strategic Air-launched cruise missile Launchers) were to be procured for the US Air Force.

October 6
First flight of an Airbus A300 with a two-man Forward Facing Crew Cockpit (FFCC). The FFCC flight deck has advanced avionics and improved system automation. This was the first time a wide-body airliner had been operated by a two-man crew.

October 9
Ascending from a site near Los Angeles, California, Fred Gorrell and John Shoecroft in the helium-filled *Superchicken III* recorded the first non-stop trans-America flight in a balloon, landing in Georgia 55hr 25min after lift-off.

October 9
Dornier began flight-testing a new four-blade propeller of advanced design. Developed by Dornier and Hoffmann, it could offer fuel savings of up to five per cent.

October 12
Aeroflot introduced the Ilyushin Il-86 wide-body jet transport on its Moscow-Prague route.

October 15
Irish commuter airline Avair took delivery of a new Shorts 330. The aircraft was used on October 26 to introduce a three-times-daily Belfast-Dublin service.

McDonnell Douglas AV-8B Harrier II.
(McDonnell Douglas)

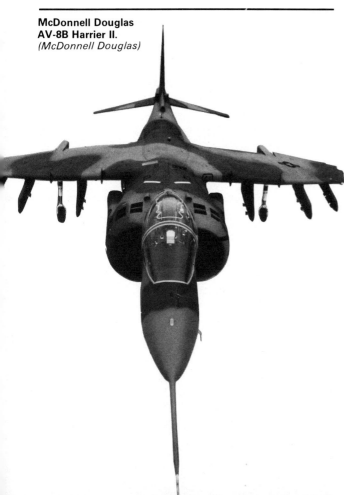

October 16
McDonnell Douglas rolled out the first full-scale development AV-8B Harrier II at St Louis, Missouri.

October 20
The Australian Minister of Defence stated that the McDonnell Douglas F-18 Hornet had been selected to meet the RAAF's tactical fighter requirement.

October 24
The Japan Air Self-Defence Force took delivery from Kawasaki of its 31st and last C-1 tactical transport.

October 30
Middle East Airlines confirmed its order for five Airbus A310s plus 14 options.

November 2
Air UK inaugurated a service linking Stansted Airport, Essex, with Amsterdam, Netherlands. This is the airport's first scheduled international service.

November 4
Second flight of Space Shuttle *Columbia* was aborted 31sec before lift-off as a result of computer problems.

November 4
The UK's Inter City Airlines (formerly Alidair) began a daily Shorts 330 service between East Midlands Airport and Brussels.

November 4
Garrett Turbine Engines began ground-testing the TFE76 engine, developed to power the US Air Force's Next Generation Trainer.

November 5
The first Lockheed Update II P-3C Orion for the Netherlands Navy was delivered to Naval Air Station Jacksonville, Florida, for initial crew training of Marine Luchtvaartdienst personnel.

November 5
The AV-8B Harrier II development aircraft made its first flight.

November 9
The first hardened aircraft shelters in the UK were put into use at RAF Honington, Suffolk.

November 12
Space Shuttle *Columbia*, carrying Joe Engle and Richard Truly, made a successful lift-off from Kennedy Space Center.

November 12
Nasa made use of two US Navy Grumman E-2C Hawkeye aircraft to monitor the Space Shuttle launch. They were intended primarily to speed tracking and recovery of the Solid Rocket Boosters (SRBs).

November 13
Ben Abruzzo, Larry Newman, Ron Clarke and Rocky Aoki completed the first manned balloon crossing of the Pacific Ocean. Carried in the helium-filled balloon *Double Eagle V*, they ended their journey from Nagashima, Japan, with a crash landing in severe

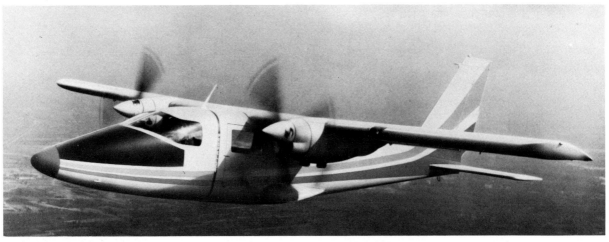

Partenavia AP.68TP. *(Aeritalia)*

weather some 148nm (274km, 170 miles) north of San Francisco.

November 14
Its mission cut short because of a fuel cell failure, Space Shuttle *Columbia* made a successful landing at Rogers Lake, Edwards AFB, California.

November 17
The Austrian Government postponed the planned procurement of 24 Dassault Mirage 50s for the nation's air force.

November 19
The US Defense Secretary announced that the British Aerospace Hawk had won the US Navy's VTX-TS trainer competition. British Aerospace and McDonnell Douglas were to be awarded contracts covering the development of the Hawk as a US Navy trainer and Sperry was to be contracted to carry out refinement of the computer software and simulators that form the ground element of VTX-TS.

November 19
The PAT-1 proof-of-concept lightplane, developed by Piper Technology Inc (no connection with Piper Aircraft Corporation), was destroyed in a flight-test accident.

November 19
The 50th anniversary of Pan American's first operation of a four-engined airliner, the Sikorsky S-40 Clipper flying boat.

November 20
The first of a production batch of 25 Partenavia AP.68TP light transport aircraft, derived from the company's P.68 Oscar, made a first flight at Naples Capodichino.

November 24
Two Sikorsky S-61Ns of Bristow Helicopters, operating in winds of about 76kt (140km/hr, 87mph), rescued 48 oilmen from the production rig *Transworld 58* after it had been blown from its North Sea moorings.

November 25
Crewed by French balloonists Hélène Dorigny and Michel Arnould, the Cameron A-530 balloon *Semiramis* (currently the world's largest hot-air balloon) flew from Ballina, Ireland, to St Christophe-en-Boucherie, France, a distance of 623nm (1,154.74km, 717.5 miles). This has since been ratified by the FAI as a new hot-air balloon distance record.

November 30
The last Westland Whirlwind helicopters on active SAR duties in the UK were retired from RAF service and replaced by the Wessex.

December 3
Aviation historian Charles Gibbs-Smith died in London following a heart attack.

December 4
Nasa accepted the first flight-standard Spacelab module at Erno's Bremen factory.

December 4
The Pakistani Government signed a letter of offer from General Dynamics covering the supply of an initial batch of six F-16s, to be delivered by December 1982.

December 5
Jerry Mullens took off in BD-2 *Phoenix*, used formerly by Jim Bede as *Love One*, for an attempt on the closed-circuit distance record for piston-engined aircraft. Landing on December 8 after 73hr 2min in the air, he had flown a distance of 8,745nm (16,206km,

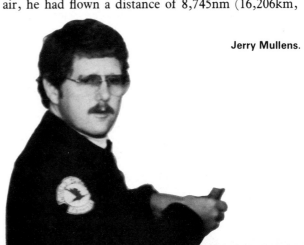

Jerry Mullens.

18

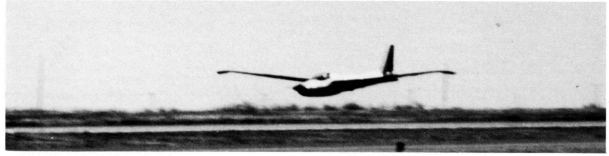

Jerry Mullens' recordbreaking *Phoenix.*

10,070 miles). Subject to ratification, this significantly exceeds the existing world record.

December 7
Lockheed stated that it intended to phase out production of the L-1011 TriStar when existing firm orders had been completed.

December 9
Aérospatiale handed over to the Armée de l'Air at Toulouse the first two of 25 new-production Transall C.160 transports.

December 11
First flight, at Reno, Nevada, of the Omac 1, the newest contender for orders in the US business aircraft market. It is also one of the most unorthodox aircraft in this category, being of canard configuration and powered by a fuselage-mounted turboprop engine driving a pusher propeller.

December 14
In a ceremony at Toulouse the Armée de l'Air accepted its 200th and last Sepecat Jaguar.

December 17
First flight, at Sandown, Isle of Wight, of the NDN 6 Fieldmaster large-capacity agricultural aircraft.

December 17
First flight of an OH-6A modified under US Army contract to NOTAR (no tail rotor) configuration. In place of a conventional anti-torque rotor the NOTAR helicopter uses pressurised air ejected through a controllable slot in the tailboom.

December 18
Dornier received German certification of its Do 228-100 15-seat utility/commuter aircraft.

December 23
A Sikorsky CH/MH-53E prototype was flown for the first time in minesweeping configuration. The US Navy plans to procure the MH-53E variant of the CH-53E heavy-lift helicopter for minesweeping duties.

December 25
Weapon Systems Operator Lt Thomas Tiller USAF was picked up from a dinghy off the North Carolina coast. He had ejected from an F-4E on December 18 and survived seven days of exposure to Atlantic conditions.

December 31
First flight of the Fairchild Swearingen Metro IIIA, a version of the Metro III powered by Pratt & Whitney Aircraft of Canada PT6A-45-6R turboprops.

1982

January 6
The aerobatic team of the Italian Air Force, the Frecce Tricolori, accepted delivery of its first Aermacchi MB.339A at Venegono airfield. The team is scheduled to receive a total of 15 MB.339As to replace its Fiat G.91s.

January 6
British Airways Helicopters accepted the first of two Westland 30s (G-BIWY). These were to be based at the airline's Beccles Heliport, Suffolk, for use in support of North Sea oil/gas platforms.

January 6
The Rolls-Royce Gem 60 turboshaft, planned to power advanced versions of the Westland 30 helicopter, began testbed running.

January 8
Air Jamaica signed a contract with Airbus Industrie for the supply of two A300B4-200s, scheduled for delivery in late 1982.

British Airways Helicopters Westland 30. *(Westland)*

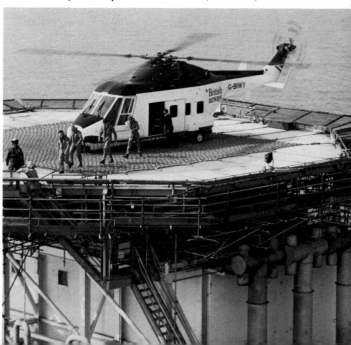

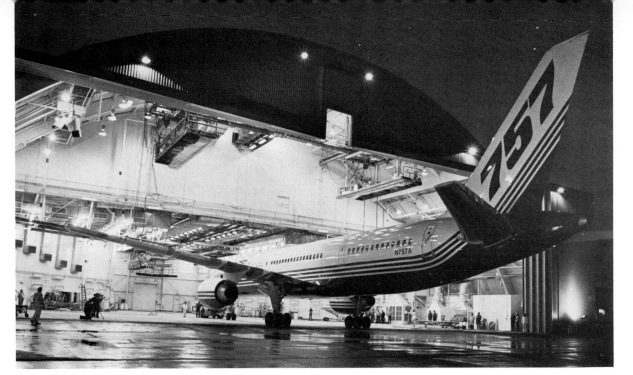

Boeing Model 757 roll-out.

January 8

A Gulfstream III executive transport operated by the US National Distillers and Chemical Corporation began a round-the-world flight. Completed on January 10, the flight, from and to Teterboro, New Jersey, was completed in 47hr 39min, breaking three existing records and setting 10 new ones.

January 13

The Kuwaiti Government concluded a $90 million contract with Lockheed-Georgia covering the supply of four L-100-30 Hercules transport aircraft for delivery to the Kuwaiti Air Force in 1983. The aircraft are needed to supplement the two L-100-20s already in service and will be used primarily for civil missions.

January 13

The first Boeing 757 twin-turbofan short/medium-range transport was rolled out at Renton, Washington.

January 14

An Algerian Air Force Lockheed C-130H located the son of British Prime Minister Margaret Thatcher in a remote region near the Mali border. The aircraft was one of two delivered during the previous month.

January 15

The first of an initial batch of 40 General Dynamics F-16 Fighting Falcons for service with the Egyptian Air Force was handed over officially at Fort Worth, Texas, with delivery to Egypt scheduled for March.

January 22

A McDonnell Douglas F-18 Hornet achieved the type's first fully automatic landing, at the Naval Air Test Center, Patuxent River, Maryland. The aircraft was controlled by an on-board autopilot linked with a ground-based SPN-42 radar.

January 22

Nato took delivery of its first Boeing E-3A Sentry Awacs aircraft at Oberpfaffenhofen. The aircraft was delivered to Geilenkirchen, West Germany, on February 24.

January 26

USAF Systems Headquarters signed a contract covering the supply of 480 General Dynamics F-16s to the US Air Force during the fiscal years 1982-85. This brought the contracted total of F-16s to 1,085, leaving only 303 of the currently planned total purchase to be negotiated.

January 27

Cessna announced the delivery of its 1,000th business jet, a Citation II. The total comprises 349 Citations, 293 Citation Is and 358 Citation IIs. First deliveries of the new Citation III were to begin in late 1982.

January 28

Hughes Helicopters flew the prototype of a new version of the Model 500. Designated Model 500E, it includes a number of improvements and a reconfigured cabin that provides more leg room for front-seat occupants.

February 4

Sikorsky operated one of the first examples of the Sikorsky S-76 II over a period of six days to set 12 new helicopter records, since ratified by the FAI. They include a helicopter speed record of 186.5kt (345.74km/hr, 214.8mph) over a 500km closed circuit, and a new altitude record in Class E-1-d of 7,940m (26,050ft).

Sikorsky S-76 II. *(Sikorsky)*

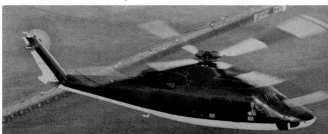

February 5
Fokker and McDonnell Douglas announced jointly that they had decided to terminate their efforts to develop the MDF-100 airliner, announced in early 1981. The recession in the commercial airliner market was cited as the primary cause for this decision.

February 6
Grob-Werke GmbH of West Germany announced a successful first flight by its G-110 two-seat lightplane. Like the Grob family of sailplanes, the G-110 is made mainly of glassfibre, and it is powered by an 88kW (118hp) Avco Lycoming O-235-M1 flat-four engine.

February 9
The Indonesian Ambassador in Paris formally accepted the first of three Transall C.160s. The first of these new-production aircraft to be sold for non-military purposes, they are to be used in transmigration flights from the heavily populated island of Java.

February 11
The Armée de l'Air accepted delivery of its 100th Alpha Jet trainer at Toulouse.

February 16
The first Airbus A310 was rolled out at Toulouse. One of the ten aircraft ordered by Swissair, this example has accommodation for 22 first-class and 190 economy-class passengers. On roll-out the A310 bore Swissair livery on one side and Lufthansa markings on the other.

February 19
The Boeing 757 made its first flight, from Renton, Washington. After 2hr 30min in the air the aircraft landed at Paine Field, where it was to be based until cleared by the FAA for operation from the company's airfield at Seattle.

February 19
The Japan Air Self-Defence Force took delivery of its 50th and last Fuji T-3 primary trainer at Utsunomiya.

February 19
The US Coast Guard took delivery of the first of 41 Dassault HU-25A Guardians.

February 22
First flight of the naval Aérospatiale SA.365F. Derived from the US Coast Guard's HH-65A, the aircraft had been modified by the company and began extensive trials with its specifically naval equipment.

Airbus A310 prototype with Lufthansa livery on one side, Swissair markings on the other. *(Airbus Industrie)*

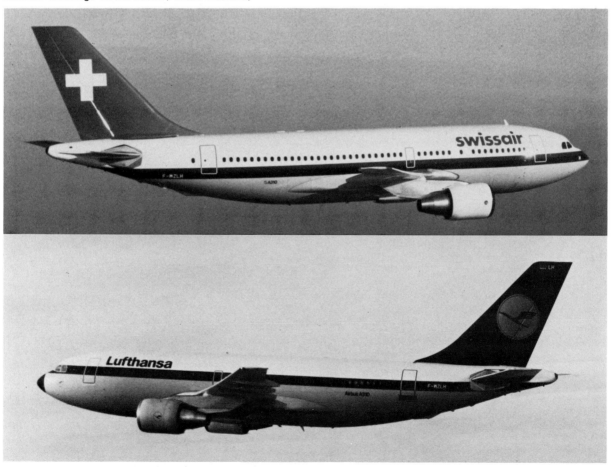

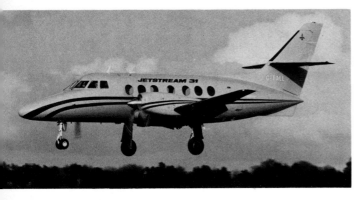

February 24

The Australian Government confirmed that it would purchase from the UK the light aircraft carrier HMS *Invincible*, which the British Government had declared surplus to requirements.

February 25

American Airlines cancelled an order for 15 Boeing 757s and options on 15 more.

February 26

Flight testing of the first production conversion of the Boeing Vertol CH-47D Chinook began at Philadelphia, Pennsylvania. The US Army planned to convert 436 CH-47As to this improved configuration, subject to satisfactory flight-test results.

March 1

The first two of 27 McDonnell Douglas F-15 Eagles to equip Alaskan Air Command arrived at Elmendorf AFB, near Anchorage. They were to replace the 21st Tactical Fighter Wing's F-4E Phantoms.

March 5

It was announced in Paris that 150 Aérospatiale TB-30 Epsilon primary trainers were to be procured for the Armée de l'Air. A first batch of 30 was to be delivered in the autumn of 1983.

March 11

Bristow Helicopters took delivery at Marignane of the first of 12 Aérospatiale AS.332L Super Pumas (G-BJXC). Bristow, which has adopted the name Tiger for these aircraft, expected to have this initial batch in service by the end of 1982. The company has 12 more on order, plus options on an additional 11.

March 12

YR-BCO, the third and last BAe One-Eleven to be assembled at Hurn for Romanian airline TAROM, was handed over, marking the end of the first phase of the manufacturing licence agreement between British Aerospace and CNIAR.

March 15

The Japan Air Self-Defence Force retired its last F-86F Sabre (62.7497). The JASDF had received a total of 479 Sabres since 1956.

March 16

First deliveries of Embraer EMB-121 Xingus for service with the French Navy and Air Force. These two forces have ordered a total of 16 and 25 respectively, to be used for aircrew training and liaison duties.

March 18

The first production British Aerospace Jetstream 31 (G-TALL) made a 1hr 5min first flight. It was anticipated that CAA certification would be gained during May 1982.

March 19

Argentinian scrap merchants landed on South Georgia to dismantle a whaling station. The Argentinian flag was flown.

March 26

Delays over funding of the Hughes AH-64A Apache Armed Attack Helicopter for the US Army came to an end with approval from the Defence System Acquisition Review Council for production of a first batch of 11 AH-64As, to be delivered in February 1984.

March 29

Brymon Airways of Plymouth, Devon, inaugurated a Plymouth-Heathrow service with a de Havilland Canada DHC-7 Dash 7.

March 31

The first Jaguar assembled by Hindustan Aeronautics made its first flight. Of the 40 new-build Jaguars being supplied by British Aerospace to the Indian Air Force, 18 had been received by the end of this month.

March 31

The 100th Panavia Tornado for the Luftwaffe (GS.018) was handed over at Manching.

April 1

The Fuerza Aerea Panamena accepted delivery at Casa's San Pablo factory of the first of three C-212 Series 200 Aviocar utility transports.

April 1

In a ceremony at Evreux, France, the Armée de l'Air's Escadron 1/64 *Béarn* took delivery of its first new-production Transall C.160 transport.

April 2

The Swedish carrier Linjeflyg AB celebrated the 25th anniversary of its formation.

April 2

Newly formed British Island Airways made its first revenue flight, from Gatwick to Catania, using BAe One-Eleven G-CIBA *Island Ensign*. An inclusive-tour operator, the company acquired its four One-Elevens from Air UK.

Bf 109 rebuilt by MBB as a Bf 109G-6. *(MBB)*

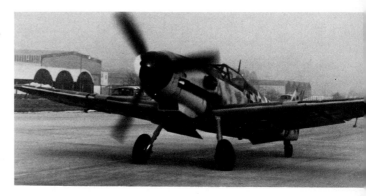

April 2
Argentinian forces invaded the Falkland Islands and, on the following day, the island of South Georgia.

April 3
The United Nations Security Council passed Resolution 502 calling for the withdrawal of Argentinian forces from the Falklands.

April 3
The first Airbus A310 (F-WZLH) made a successful first flight of 3hr 15min at Toulouse.

April 5
The main elements of the British Task Force for operations against the Argentinian forces on the Falklands sailed from Portsmouth. They included the carriers HMS *Hermes* and *Invincible*.

April 6
A new Sea Harrier squadron, No 809, was formed at RNAS Yeovilton.

April 7
The British Government declared a 200-mile exclusion zone around the Falkland Islands.

April 10
First flight of the Canadair CL-601 Challenger. This version differs from the standard Challenger 600 in having 38.48kN (8,650lb st) General Electric CF34-1A turbofans and wingtip winglets.

April 21
Two Westland Wessex helicopters of the British Task Force crashed on South Georgia in bad weather. A third recovered the crews and the men of the SAS who were aboard the first two.

April 23
First flight of the Bf 109 rebuilt by Messerschmitt-Bölkow-Blohm. Configured as a Bf 109G-6 and registered D-FMBB, it combines the airframe of a Hispano licence-built HA.1112 (c/n 195) with a Swedish licence-built Daimler-Benz DB 605 engine (s/n 2293).

April 25
Aircraft attached to the British Task Force despatched to the Falkland Islands were in action for the first time. Lynx helicopters flying from the frigates HMS *Alacrity* and *Antelope* attacked the Argentine submarine *Santa Fe* off Grytviken harbour, South Georgia. Later that day Sea Kings escorted by Lynxes landed Royal Marines on South Georgia. The Marines subsequently recaptured the island from the Argentinian land force.

April 28
The British Government gave Argentina 48hr warning that an air blockade would be imposed over a 200-mile (322km) radius from the Falklands.

May 1
The first British air attack against Argentinian positions on the Falkland Islands was made by a single Vulcan B2 operating from Ascension Island. This called for flight refuelling on both the outward and return flights. The Vulcan bombed Port Stanley airfield, and an attack on the same target was made immediately afterwards by nine Sea Harriers from HMS *Hermes*. Three Sea Harriers also attacked the airstrip at Goose Green. All aircraft returned safely. The Vulcan operation against Port Stanley from Ascension Island must rank as the RAF's longest operational sortie.

May 1
In the first Sea Harrier combat victory against Argentinian aircraft a Mirage IIIEA was destroyed by a Sidewinder missile. A Mirage III and a Canberra bomber were lost in other engagements on the same day.

May 2
A Royal Navy ASW Sea King came under fire from the Argentine patrol vessel *Alferez Sobral* and reported its position to the Task Force. Shortly afterwards the *Sobral* was severely damaged in an attack by two Lynx helicopters deploying Sea Skua missiles. An accompanying patrol vessel, the *Comodoro Somellera*, was sunk.

May 2
The Argentinian Navy cruiser *General Belgrano* was sunk by a British nuclear-powered submarine. A total of 382 sailors lost their lives but many more were rescued.

May 4
In an air attack on the British task force an Exocet missile fired from a Super Etendard of the Argentinian Navy hit the Type 42 destroyer HMS *Sheffield*. Severe fire resulted in the *Sheffield* being abandoned, and she subsequently sank during bad weather. Twenty sailors lost their lives.

May 4
A Sea Harrier was lost during an attack on Port Stanley.

May 5
Two British Airways L-1011 TriStars achieved safe

touchdowns at London's Heathrow Airport in totally blind conditions. The landings were made in the absence of reference height and runway visual range measurements.

May 7
The British Government declared a "safe zone" extending 12 miles from the Argentinian coast.

May 7
A new Sea King squadron, No 825, was commissioned at RNAS Culdrose.

May 7
Two Sea Harriers from HMS *Invincible* were lost. They are believed to have collided in poor visibility.

May 8
Sea Harriers prevented transport aircraft from bringing in reinforcements and supplies for the Argentinian forces on the Falklands.

May 8
About 20 Harriers and Sea Harriers flew non-stop from RNAS Yeovilton to Ascension Island. They were air-refuelled several times during the 9hr flight.

May 9
The Argentinian vessel *Narwal*, which had been shadowing the British task force, was attacked by two Sea Harriers. The crew subsequently surrendered to a boarding party from HMS *Hermes*.

May 13
Soyuz T-5 was launched successfully from Baikonur, carrying cosmonauts Anatoli Berezovoy and Valentin Lebedev. A successful link-up was made on May 14 with the Soviet Union's new orbiting laboratory, Salyut 7.

May 14
The British Task Force raided Pebble Island. Three Argentinian Skyhawk bombers were lost in action.

May 15
India's combined communications and weather satellite, Insat 1A, became operational after a Delta launch into Earth orbit during April.

May 17
In what is believed to be the first launch of a satellite from an orbiting space station, the crew of Salyut 7 placed the amateur radio satellite Iskra 2 in Earth orbit by means of an airlock in the space laboratory.

May 19
Space Shuttle *Columbia* was moved into the Vehicle Assembly Building for mating of the Orbiter with the External Tank and SRBs. This was in preparation for *Columbia*'s fourth mission, then scheduled to begin on June 27.

May 21
Royal Marine Commandos and a Parachute Regiment battalion made a successful landing at Port San Carlos on the East Falklands. Royal Navy Sea King HC4s played a major role in these operations.

May 21
HMS *Ardent*, a Type 21 frigate, was lost after an air attack. British troops established a beach-head at San Carlos. Nine Argentinian aircraft were lost in action.

May 24
The last Boeing 707 in operation with British Airways made its final flight, from Cairo to London Heathrow. The type had been in service with BOAC/British Airways since 1960.

May 24
Following several hits by rockets and bombs launched from Argentinian aircraft on May 23, the frigate HMS *Antelope* of the British Task Force blew up and sank. Seven Argentinian aircraft were lost in action.

May 25
The Type 42 destroyer HMS *Coventry* of the British Task Force was hit by bombs from Argentinian Skyhawks and caught fire. She later capsized and sank. In another attack on the same day the container ship *Atlantic Conveyor* was hit by an Exocet missile launched from an Argentinian Navy Super Etendard. The vessel caught fire and was abandoned. Twenty-four Task Force personnel lost their lives.

May 28
Goose Green and Darwin were retaken by British forces. Seventeen British soldiers lost their lives.

June 3
An RAF Vulcan was intercepted in Brazilian airspace and escorted to Rio de Janeiro by Brazilian F-5Es.

June 6
Backed by extensive air strikes, Israeli armour and troops invaded southern Lebanon.

June 8
Argentinian aircraft attacked Task Force ships at Bluff Cove, resulting in heavy loss of life. Eleven Argentinian aircraft were lost in action.

June 12
HMS *Glamorgan* was struck by a land-based Exocet fired from Port Stanley. Thirteen sailors were lost but the destroyer remained operational.

June 14
Argentinian forces on the Falklands surrendered. Their losses amounted to more than 700 killed, five ships and more than 100 aircraft. British air losses in action totalled 10 Harriers and Sea Harriers and a number of helicopters, including one Sea King that crashed in Chile. No Harrier or Sea Harrier was lost in air-to-air combat.

June 22
First flight of the BAe VC10 K2 flight-refuelling tanker for the RAF.

The Incredible Harrier

REGINALD TURNILL

" ...the incredible efforts of the Harrier." — Cdr Chris Craig, HMS *Alacrity*, at the end of the Falklands War

"The Sea Harrier has been absolutely superb." — Capt L. C. Middleton, HMS *Hermes*

"Developing the Harrier has been a 25-year battle, and at times it looked like a losing battle." — John Fozard, Harrier chief designer

"I felt a great responsibility when the Task Force set off for the Falklands, because without the Harrier and the air cover it provided I do not think they would have gone ....We can all stick our chests out with pride." — Sir Stanley Hooker, designer of the Pegasus engine

Whether it will ever be officially admitted seems doubtful. But the fact is that recovery of the Falkland Islands

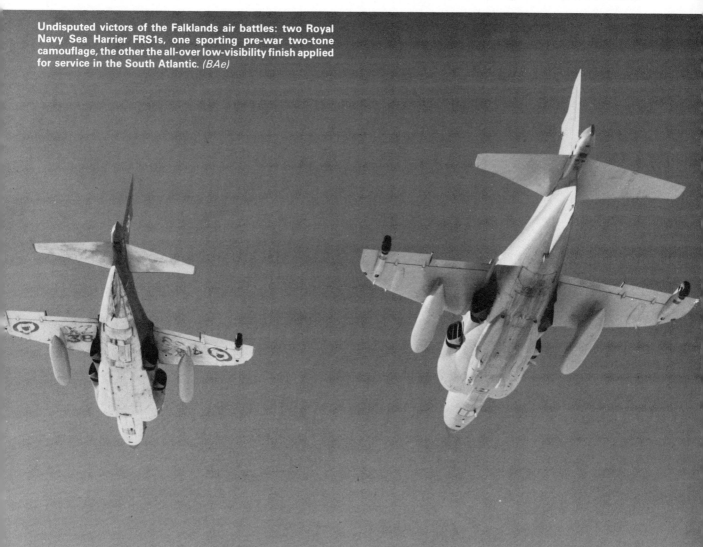

Undisputed victors of the Falklands air battles: two Royal Navy Sea Harrier FRS1s, one sporting pre-war two-tone camouflage, the other the all-over low-visibility finish applied for service in the South Atlantic. *(BAe)*

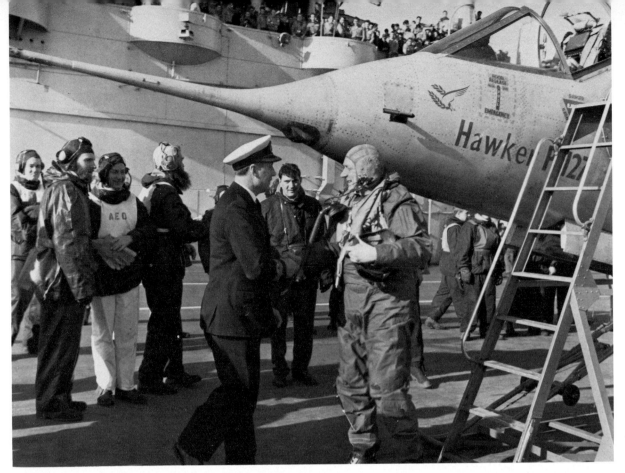

The man and the aircraft that started it all: Bill Bedford and the Hawker P.1127 on the flight deck of HMS *Ark Royal* after the type's first ever shipboard landing, carried out on February 8, 1963.

would not have been possible without the Harrier. The Navy's Task Force could not have survived as well as it did without the air cover — limited though it was — that they provided. No other British aircraft could have done the job in those conditions. Without these unique aircraft, therefore, it is certain that the Defence Staff would never have agreed to the Task Force being sent.

During the 10-week confrontation between Britain and Argentina defence organisations around the world focused on it to see what lessons they could learn: had they bought the right equipment for their own services, and would they be able to use it effectively and efficiently if they encountered a similar crisis? British Aerospace, whose Kingston, Surrey/Brough, Yorkshire Division builds the Harrier, has had a nostalgia-provoking reminder of what things used to be like for Britain's aerospace industry, with international defence experts beating a path to their office doors seeking performance details of the missiles and aircraft locked in battle in the South Atlantic.

The situation had equal fascination for aerospace correspondents. For 25 years Britain's development of V/Stol, and particularly of the Harrier, has been one of three main threads running through the period (the others being Concorde and spaceflight). As each day brought news of fresh Harrier successes, punctuated by announcements of the inevitable losses, my thoughts frequently turned to the men whose persistence throughout those years had ensured that once again, when war came, Britain had the right aircraft for the occasion. Some people, arguing that nobody could have foreseen the Falklands situation, might call it luck. It was no such thing.

Disastrous early days

Since the original Hawker Siddeley P.1127 was first test-flown from RAE Farnborough by Bill Bedford in March 1961, I had covered his demonstrations, and interviewed him afterwards for BBC radio and TV, countless times. I remembered him grey with fatigue and momentarily close to despair after having to eject in December 1961, and after crashing at the Paris Salon in June 1963.

I remembered too the men behind him and the Harrier for all those years, starting with engineer Ralph Hooper, responsible for the original creative design in 1957, followed by John Fozard, chief Harrier designer from 1965, and Sir Stanley Hooker, whose Bristol Siddeley Pegasus engine with its swivelling nozzles had made it all possible.

A few days after the final Falklands triumph I went to see Bill Bedford, now 61 and British Aerospace's marketing manager special projects, at his Kingston office. He was surprisingly subdued. Half jokingly, I asked whether anybody had suggested sending him to the South Atlantic to help brief the Harrier pilots. "I'm an old-generation aviator now," he said. "I have to let the youngsters get on with it. They know much more than I do nowadays — and I have to be careful I don't get too egotistical. But it's a fact that for much of its life the Harrier has been a misunderstood and much maligned aeroplane. So it's tremendous to have been involved with a project like this, to have seen it in operational use at last, and to feel that some of the things we have said it can do in the past have at last been proved by what it has actually done. But when you are in the sharp end of the plane, you sit in the hot seat, and the spotlight shines on you rather disproportionately and a little unfairly. There are so many other people involved: very good pilots, for instance, like Hugh Merewether, who worked for me like the current test pilots under John Farley, himself one of the greatest test pilots the country has ever had."

Pictured together at a time when their Falklands baptism of fire still lay ahead, HMS *Invincible* **and five Sea Harriers of No 801 Sqn formate briefly for the publicity cameras.** *(BAe)*

The Harrier's Falklands tally

When I saw Bill Bedford, British Aerospace was still short of detailed information about how the Task Force Harriers had been used in combat and exactly how they had accounted for at least 28 enemy aircraft, though most were known to have been shot down by AIM-9L Sidewinder missiles, with five or more falling to cannon fire. But he produced with pride a letter scribbled during the action by Captain Lyn Middleton RN, in command of HMS *Hermes*, saying: "I know you and the boys in the factory would want to know that the Sea Harrier has been absolutely superb. The serviceability has been astonishingly good: after a hard day's/night's flying, we never seem to have less than 80 per cent serviceable. In air combat we have not lost an aircraft."

A telex had also arrived from the Ministry of Defence: "The Sea Harriers dominated the air-defence battle. No Sea Harriers were lost in air-to-air combat, and their weapon system was entirely a success. Serviceability of the aircraft and weapon systems was high

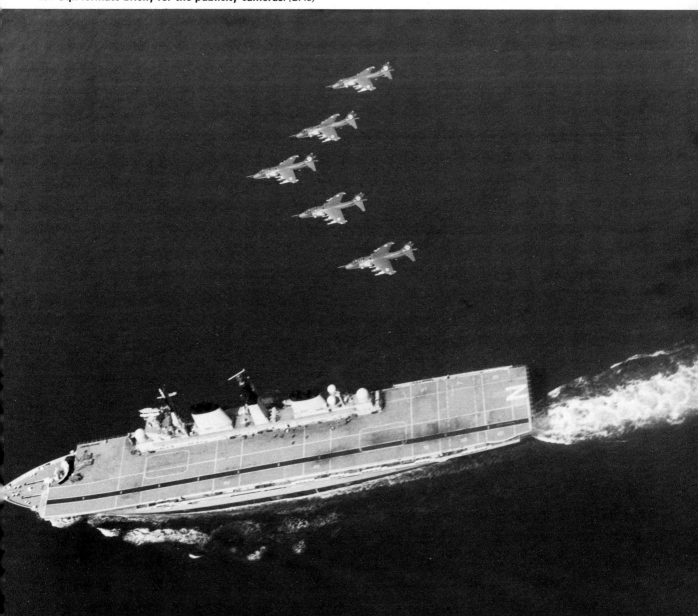

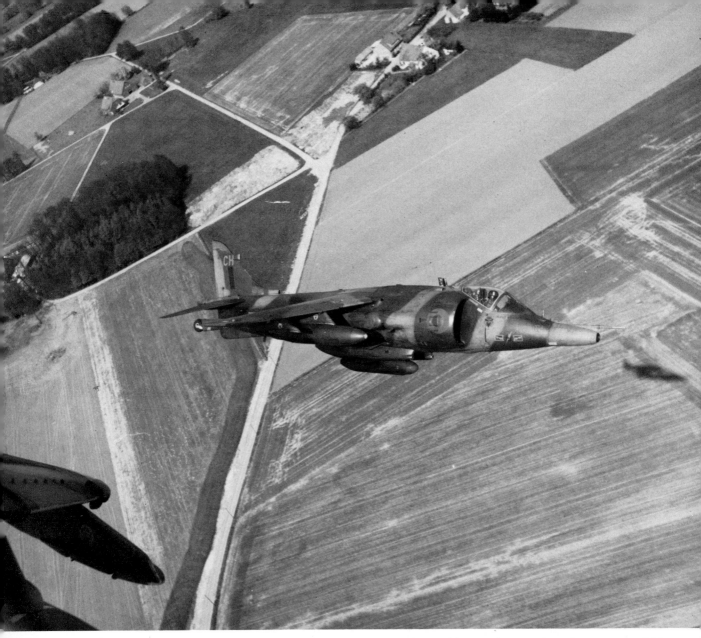

The RAF's Harrier GR3 was the Sea Harrier's comrade-in-arms during the Falklands campaign, taking over the ground-attack role and freeing the naval aircraft for the vital task of air defence. *(Crown Copyright)*

throughout. The Sea Harrier and Harrier demonstrated added flexibility by using air-to-air refuelling to allow them to be deployed direct from the UK. During the operations, both within the open waters in the Total Exclusion Zone, and also over the coastal waters around the Falkland Islands, the Sea Harrier accounted for 20 Mirage and A-4 aircraft, as well as a number of Pucaras, Hercules, Canberras, helicopters, etc."

It was the 80 per cent serviceability that gave Bill Bedford most satisfaction. "In the past a lot of people have shaken their heads over the alleged complications of the Harrier, with its vectoring of thrust. In fact, as we have pointed out, vectoring does not add to complexity at all; in its avionics it's no different from any

other plane with a modern nav/attack system, and it's very reliable. The RAF Harriers from Wittering flew to Ascension in 9½hr, and then on to the Task Force from there: a total flight of 17hr. At the end of that some of the pilots made their first ever landing on a ship at sea — a vertical landing, of course. That's indicative of the flexibility of the little aeroplane."

Operating to the limit

Bill invariably speaks of "aeroplanes" rather than "aircraft" and of the Harrier as "the little aeroplane". Every time I heard a loss reported, I told him, I was worried because I knew the Task Force had so few Harriers. "They were operating to the limit in a hostile environment," he said quietly. "Imagine the pitching and heaving and rolling of the ships, with icing, poor visibility and low cloudbase; in a situation like that you are bound to lose a few, aren't you?" One cannot help wondering how many more ships the Navy might have lost if the Harriers completing the last leg of their

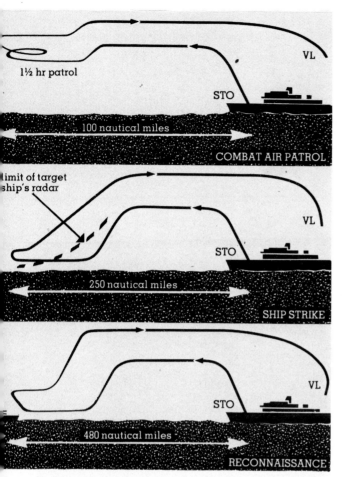

1½ hr patrol

VL

STO

100 nautical miles

COMBAT AIR PATROL

limit of target ship's radar

VL

STO

250 nautical miles

SHIP STRIKE

VL

STO

480 nautical miles

RECONNAISSANCE

Designed for operation from small carriers accommodating no more than a dozen fixed-wing aircraft, the Sea Harrier makes up for lack of numbers with its versatility. For a standard CAP mission it is equipped with pairs of AIM-9L Sidewinder air-to-air missiles, 30mm Aden cannon, and drop tanks. Principal weapon for ship strikes will be the BAe Sea Eagle air-to-surface missile. For reconnaissance the type has a built-in nose-mounted oblique camera and can carry a five-camera pod on the underfuselage pylon. *(BAe)*

journey to the Falklands aboard *Atlantic Conveyor* had gone down with it, instead of having been flown off before it was hit by an Exocet missile.

Both Bill Bedford and John Fozard were repeatedly asked how it was that the subsonic Harrier could so successfully shoot down the supersonic Mirage. "What few people realise," said Bill, "is that the Harrier has got the climb and acceleration of a supersonic plane because it has a tremendously high thrust-to-weight ratio. Fuel consumption is relatively low when flying at maximum thrust because it is a non-reheated power-plant; therefore in combat missions the Harrier pilot is not going to be quite so embarrassed about a shortage of fuel as the opposition will be, operating with reheat. A Mirage using afterburning at low level consumes three to four times the fuel per minute that a Harrier uses in combat. In simulated dogfights carried out by the US Marines against F-14s, the Harrier almost invariably

prevented the F-14 from staying on its tail. That doesn't mean to say it would not have got shot down; but in three minutes the F-14 used 6,000lb of fuel, the Harrier only 600lb. Interesting ratio, isn't it? Another good thing in favour of the Harrier is that it's small and very difficult to see, with low smoke emission as well. And perhaps the most important factor of all is the ability to vector thrust in flight: the pilot can produce abrupt deceleration and rapid manoeuvre initiation, forcing the attacking aeroplane to overshoot; that enables the Harrier to change from being the attacked to the attacker."

To the outside observer, perhaps the most incredible feature of the Harrier story in the Falklands is the warmth of the tributes to its usefulness from the service which for so long resolutely rejected it as being much too limited for naval use. Bill Bedford explained it like this: "We always thought the aeroplane provided the fundamental elements which are so important for winning wars: mobility, flexibility and surprise. For land operations large airfields weren't required, hence Harriers could operate from the modest facilities available in the Falklands. The naval application was always a potential in our minds, but it was only natural that in the early 1960s the Navy chiefs were fighting hard for the big ship. In an ideal world they would have liked the higher performance — bigger warload, greater radius of action, supersonics — and all the other benefits obtainable from conventional aircraft operation from carriers. This could not be directly replaced with the V/Stol generation we had at that time. But the defence budgets were cut by successive governments, and the large ships were finally discarded. But even then it took quite a long time to get the doubting Thomases fully behind the Sea Harrier, which was not finally delivered into service until June 1979. That *is* a long time, isn't it?"

Unmatched versatility

The varied roles performed by the Sea Harrier include air defence, patrolling for over 1½hr at 100 nautical miles from the ship; reconnaissance and probe for surface ships using Blue Fox, the radar warning receiver and cameras; and strike/ground attack on ship and shore targets with a wide variety of ordnance and stand-off air-to-surface missiles. The Harrier's unique ability to refuel on the aft platform of small ships steaming well forward of the carriers was used in the Falklands crisis. This is analogous to the RAF and US Marine Corps' dispersed-site forward basing on land.

But despite their confidence in those early days in the long-term potential of V/Stol, Bill Bedford admitted he had never dreamed of the feature that is now an essential adjunct of naval operations with the type: the Ski-jump, which played a major part in the Harrier's South Atlantic triumph. The principle was originally proposed by a Royal Navy engineer, Lt Cdr Doug Taylor, in

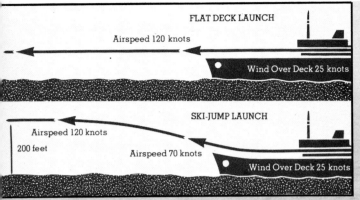

FLAT DECK LAUNCH

Airspeed 120 knots

Wind Over Deck 25 knots

SKI-JUMP LAUNCH

Airspeed 120 knots

200 feet

Airspeed 70 knots

Wind Over Deck 25 knots

Latest in a line of British developments that have revolutionised naval aviation, the brilliantly simple Ski-jump transforms the Sea Harrier's payload/range performance and reduces the risks of the launch. Below A Sea Harrier goes ballistic from the deck of HMS *Invincible*. Left The perform-ance benefits of Ski-jump. Launching from a 600ft flat deck into a 25kt wind, Sea Harrier can carry a 10,000lb load of fuel and weapons. Fit a 15° Ski-jump and under the same condi-tions the aircraft can take off with 30 per cent more useful load. *(BAe)*

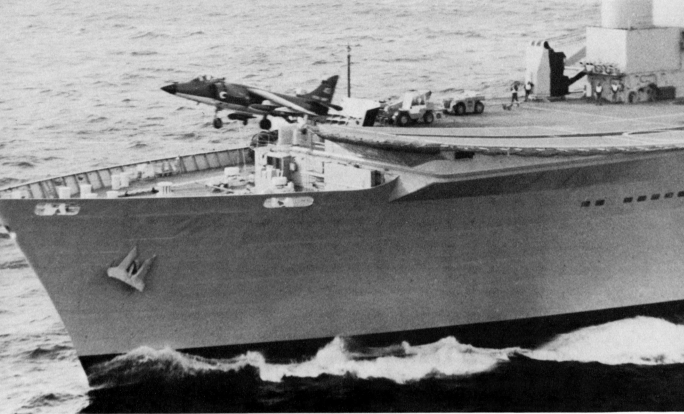

For the Harrier, home is any flat, reasonably firm and stable spot. During the Falklands campaign Harriers landed on and took off from container ships and frigate and destroyer helicopter decks. *(BAe)*

a thesis presented at Southampton University in 1973. His wife was an enthusiastic skier, and study of the effects of ski-jumps on a downward track gave him the idea of doing it the other way round. The semi-ballistic trajectory afforded by the 7° ramp on HMS *Invincible* and the 12° ramp on HMS *Hermes* allows the Harrier to take off with well over 2,500lb (1,100kg) more fuel or weapons than from a flat deck, or alternatively shortens the take-off run by up to 60 per cent. In all cases it increases safety by making the entire launch sequence simpler and easier for the pilot.

It was on February 8, 1963, that Bill Bedford carried out the landing that 19 years later made the Harrier's performance in the Falklands possible. He made the first vertical landing on HMS *Ark Royal*'s flight deck,

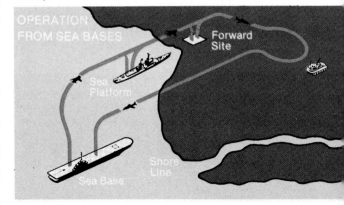

OPERATION FROM SEA BASES

Forward Site

Sea Platform

Shore Line

Sea Base

followed by a series of short take-offs, and he recalls Admiral Donald Gibson saying that what had impressed him was the complete absence of fright on the faces of the spectators. New aircraft normally thundered aboard aircraft carriers bigger, heavier and faster, and here at last was a reversal of the trend. "We proved that landlubbers could readily operate jet V/Stol planes from a ship without very specialised training, and that it was so much easier than trying to land a conventional aeroplane on a ship," said Bill.

But although they gave Bill his naval wings as a result, the Royal Navy was then operating the Buccaneer and Sea Vixen, and eyeing America's Phantom, which was later procured. "They looked on V/Stol with interest, but a certain amount of suspicion. It was still a bit early in the day for them, really".

Cancellations not all bad

It must have been an awful shock when, two years later, Defence Minister Denis Healey announced the cancellation of the P.1154, the supersonic version of what later became the subsonic Harrier, and of the TSR.2 and the Armstrong Whitworth 681 V/Stol transport. But looking back, I suspect that both Bill Bedford and John Fozard would probably agree that the cancellations, accompanied as they were by a subsonic version of the Harrier being imposed upon the Navy, had in the end turned out rather well from their point of view. In those more competitive days — long before the rival British planemakers had finally been merged into one group — they did tend to oversell the Harrier. It seems very unlikely at this stage that a supersonic Harrier would have done any better in the Falklands; on the contrary, a heavier, more complex aircraft might not have done nearly so well. Several times in subsequent years even the subsonic Harrier came up again for possible cancellation in defence reviews, and rumour has it that in 1967 it was Jim Callaghan's support in Cabinet that finally enabled it to escape the axe and enter RAF service in 1969.

Now, 15 years later, as John Fozard points out, the Sea Harrier has shown the world that it is possible to reverse the hitherto unbroken trend towards bigger and more expensive ships and weapon systems. Even ships like HMS *Invincible*, it can be argued, are too big for Harrier. Effective air power at sea, incorporating strike, reconnaissance and fighter capability, is available with cheaper, more affordable ships. The work done on the cancelled P.1154 all those years ago will not be wasted. The design team of the 1960s learned a lot from their plans for a 30,000lb-thrust Pegasus engine using plenum chamber burning, in which the gases from the burnt fuel were expelled from the front nozzles to provide the higher gas velocities and temperatures necessary for supersonic flight. Now that design experience is backed with vast operational experience of subsonic V/Stol on land and at sea.

The US Marine Corps is known to feel that the Falklands War has more than justified its decision to go ahead with building 336 AV-8B Harrier IIs, or Harrier GR5s as they are known to the RAF, which has ordered 60. Bill Bedford thinks that the whole exercise will act as a "ski-jump" for the supersonic Harrier needed for the 1990s and developed by British Aerospace as a collaborative programme, probably with the United States and perhaps with European partners as well.

The Harrier in Combat

About 40 Harriers were used in the Falklands War, of which ten were lost. There were only 20 available aboard HMS *Hermes* and HMS *Invincible* when the Task Force first arrived. But that "handful of aircraft," in the words of an RN captain, quickly established air superiority over 200 enemy Mirage IIIs and 5s and A-4 Skyhawks. The Sea Harriers shot down 28 enemy aircraft and lost none themselves in air combat, though during the campaign seven aircraft and four pilots were lost to other causes. RAF Harrier GR3s flew 150 operational sorties, successfully attacking ground targets at Port Stanley and elsewhere; three aircraft were shot down but all the pilots ejected and survived.

Sea Harriers

1 slid off *Hermes'* deck when attempting to land after being damaged by ground fire. Pilot recovered.

1 exploded during take-off either from *Hermes* or *Invincible*; pilot killed.

1 ditched after being damaged by ground fire over Port Stanley; pilot recovered after nine hours in dinghy.

2 lost either by colliding or flying into sea when being vectored on to a suspected target. Both pilots killed.

1 shot down over Goose Green. Pilot killed.

1 brought down by ground fire (probably a Shorts Blowpipe). Ft Lt Jeffrey Glover ejected with broken arm and other injuries, was captured and taken to Argentina. The only British POW, he was released on July 9, 1982.

(One Sea Harrier was also lost at RNAS Yeovilton during ski-jump exercises. Pilot ejected safely).

RAF Harrier GR3s

3 brought down by ground fire but all pilots ejected safely. Sqn Ldr Bob Iverson ejected during advance on Port Stanley and was recovered by helicopter after sheltering for two nights in a deserted farmhouse.

Harrier facts

First flights

Variant	First flight		Serial No
	Tethered	**Conventional**	
P.1127	October 21, 1960	March 13, 1961	XP831
Kestrel	—	March 7, 1964	XS688
Harrier GR1/3 (P.1127 [RAF])	—	August 31, 1966	XV276
Harrier T2/4	—	April 24, 1969	XW174
AV-8A	—	November 20, 1970	158384
Harrier Mk 52	—	September 16, 1971	G-VTOL
TAV-8A	—	July 16, 1975	159378
AV-8S Matador	—	September 18, 1975	159560
TAV-8S	—	February 25, 1976	159563
Sea Harrier FRS1	—	August 20, 1978	XZ450
YAV-8B	—	November 9, 1978	158394
AV-8B Harrier II	—	November 5, 1981	161396
Harrier GR5 (projected)	—	early 1984	

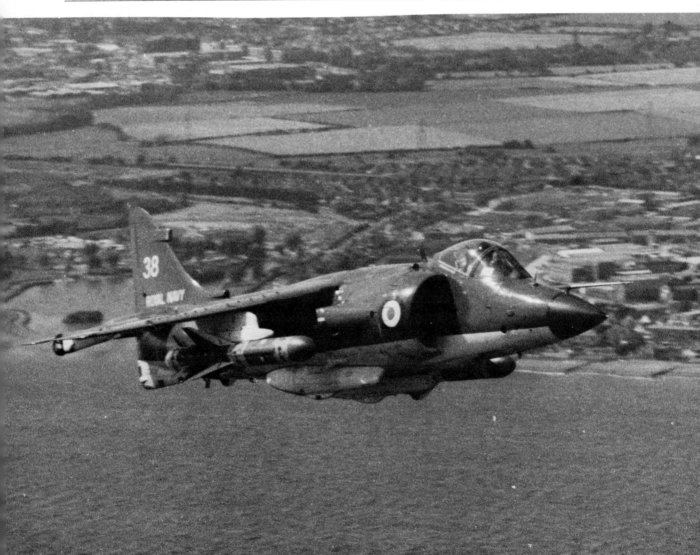

Order book

Operator	Variant	Single-seat	Two-seat	
RAF	P.1127	6	—	—
RAF	Kestrel	9	—	—
RAF	GR1/3	120	T2/4	23
RAF	GR5	60	—	—
US Marine Corps	AV-8A	102	TAV-8A	8
US Marine Corps	AV-8B	336	—	—
Spanish Navy	AV-8S	11	TAV-8S	2
Royal Navy	FRS1	48	T4	4
Indian Navy	FRS51	6	T60	2
British Aerospace		—	Mk 52	1
Totals		**698**		**40**

Export mark numbers

50	USMC AV-8A
51	Indian Navy Sea Harrier FRS
52	BAe demonstrator (G-VTOL)
53	
54	USMC TAV-8A
55	Spanish Navy AV-8S
56	
57	
58	Spanish Navy TAV-8S
59	
60	Indian Navy two-seater

Production aircraft first delivery dates

P.1127	(test only)
Kestrel	June 1964
Harrier GR1	April 1968
Harrier T2	July 1970
AV-8A	January 1971
TAV-8A	October 1975
Matador	November 1975
Sea Harrier	June 1979
AV-8B (projected)	November 1983
Harrier GR5 (projected)	mid-1986

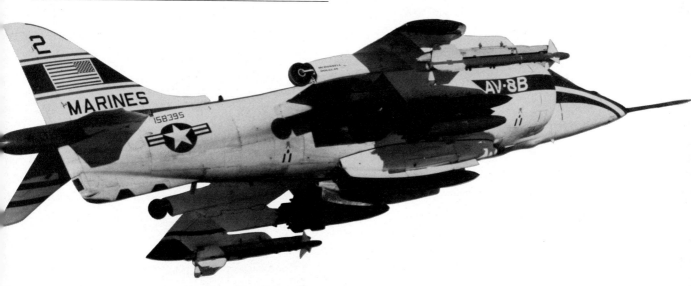

Above **One of the two AV-8As modified to serve as AV-8B prototypes. The Harrier development initiative has now passed to the United States, where McDonnell Douglas is tooling up for production of the AV-8B Harrier II. Can Britain regain control of its own creation by taking the lead on a supersonic Harrier for the 1990s?** *(McDonnell Douglas)*

Left **Sea Harrier carrying trial rounds of the Sea Eagle anti-ship missile, a combination that is likely to prove even more lethal than the Super Etendard/Exocet, used to such effect against the Falklands Task Force.** *(BAe)*

The Royal Navy's newest Sea Harrier squadron, No 809, lined up in parade order at home base RNAS Yeovilton. (BAe)

Wings for the Third World

JOHN W. R. TAYLOR

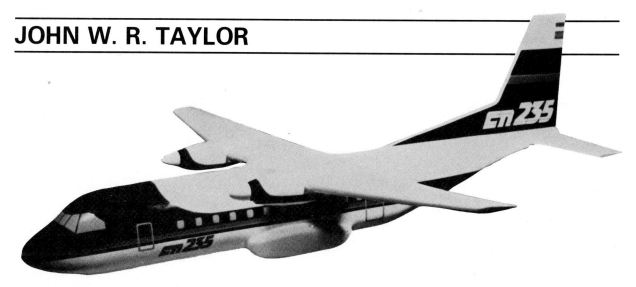

Model of the CN-235 twin-turboprop transport, under joint development by CASA of Spain and Nurtanio of Indonesia.

The aircraft salesman from Western Europe, hoping to build on earlier successes in Jakarta, had no doubts concerning the fate of the four or five new airliners that would soon be competing for orders in the 30/40-seat category. One of them was little more than a glint in its designer's eye. Two others were products of still new industries in Third World countries, off the edges of the map on the walls of people who bought airliners in quantity .... Within a minute or two the contenders had been whittled down to a single type "which could not fail," being a product of two of the most experienced and respected national consortia in the world, working in partnership. But was the salesman correct?

Fifteen minutes before this gratuitous exposé of the prospects for the future wellbeing of worldwide aircraft manufacturers, the writer had benefitted from a briefing by the president of Indonesia's domestic airline, Merpati Nusantara. He anticipated a need for at least 100 of the CN-235 twin-turboprop 34/38-seaters being developed by his nation's own aircraft manufacturer, Nurtanio Aircraft Industry, at Bandung in collaboration with CASA of Spain.

Indonesia consists of 13,677 islands and islets with an estimated total population of 150 million. Too many of them live on Java, so the government has instituted a transmigration scheme under which family groups from overpopulated regions can move voluntarily to new homes on the smaller islands. In the first year and a half of the operation more than 200,000 people were relocated by three of a growing fleet of "stretched" Lockheed L-100-30 Hercules transports. Well over a million people will eventually take advantage of the transmigration airlift. Merpati Nusantara will then help to ensure that they are kept supplied with everything needed to make a success of their new lives, and that they never feel cut off from old friends and surroundings.

The scale of even routine air transportation in Indonesia is evident from a glance at the operating statistics of Merpati. By February 1982 its six Viscounts had each logged between 32,268 and 41,697 flying hours. One of its F.27s was nudging 54,700 hours, involving 58,345 landings. How can anyone predict an uncertain future for an aircraft as promising as the CN-235, built in a nation with such a clear demand for aerial buses and trucks?

What Indonesia, and the rest of the Third World, does not need is Western-style sophistication. Aircraft have to be sturdy, reliable and able to operate into small, remote places with limited ground facilities. This makes life a little easier for a manufacturer like Nurtanio. Less apparent, except to a visitor to Bandung, are the advantages inherent in the environment and in a large domestic market. Requiring a new fac-

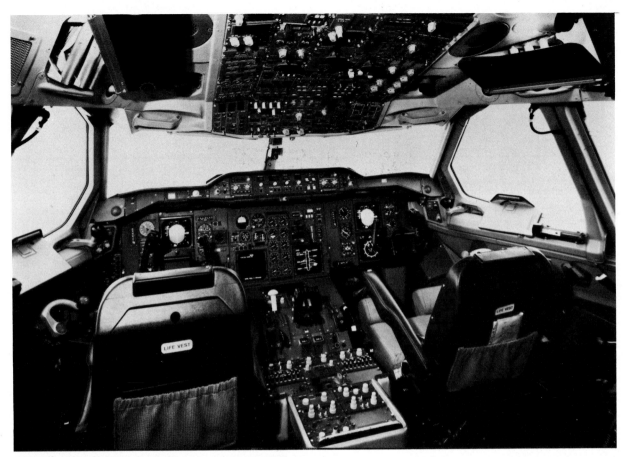

The forward-facing crew cockpit proposed by Mr Wiweko Soepono of Garuda Indonesian Airlines will be standard on the Airbus A310, shown here. *(Airbus Industrie)*

tory nine times the size of its original works in which to produce the CN-235 simultaneously with other fixed-wing aircraft and helicopters, Nurtanio broke ground for a 38.5-hectare (95-acre) administration, manufacturing, welfare and recreational complex in mid-1980. Within 18 months components for the CN-235 were coming off rows of immaculate computer-controlled machines in its halls. Quality is high, and operating costs are lower than elsewhere because no artificial factory lighting or heating are needed at the near-equatorial latitude of Java.

Such natural benefits help to offset remoteness from sources of equipment and a genuine shortness of funds. Thus, while airlines like Braniff in the USA and Laker in the UK have been forced out of business during the past year by muddled deregulation and the cheap-fare war, operators like Garuda of Indonesia grow healthier as a result of a more simple and practical approach to some of the same objectives.

Needing to provide rock-bottom fares for Moslems making their long pilgrimage of a lifetime from Jakarta to Mecca, Garuda discovered that without sacrifice of safety standards it could seat an unprecedented 542 passengers in a Boeing 747. Only a negative response to enquiries addressed to a somewhat startled Boeing scuttled a proposal to install further seats and lighting in the cargo holds for passengers who seldom have much baggage. Such ideas, peculiar to realistic Third World thinking, should never be mistaken for technological naivety. Mr Wiweko Soepono, the dynamic president director of Garuda who packages pilgrims so economically in 747s, was also responsible for the year's major contribution to economy in big-time airline operations.

For years airline pilots' organisations have tried to convince their employers and the licensing authorities that three pilots are essential on the flight deck to ensure the safe, efficient operation of a big jet. That fine old English author of country books, A. G. Street, always claimed that one boy on a farm does a boy's work, whereas two boys do half a boy's work and three do no work at all. Nobody would pretend that such a scurrilous view applies also to triplicated drivers of aircraft, but there is little to suggest that a third pilot makes flying safer. With this in mind, and with long experience as a transport pilot influencing his thoughts at least as much as did his presidency of Garuda, Mr Wiweko envisaged what is now known as the forward-facing crew cockpit (FFCC).

Reduced to simple terms, when three pilots are carried by a modern airliner two of them face forward and the third sideways at what used to be the flight engineer's station. With the FFCC, the instruments and controls that were formerly on the side panel are transferred to the front of the cockpit so that everything can be monitored and controlled by a two-man crew. There is provision for a training or check pilot, if required, between and behind the pilots. More important, the latest concepts in CRT technology and colour-coded push-button selectors/indicators are used to provide better and clearer information on forward and overhead panels, so reducing the pilots' workload.

The first operational FFCC was worked out in partnership by Mr Wiweko and engineers at Airbus Industrie for standard installation on the A300 transports owned by Garuda. Within months the idea had gained such acceptance that Boeing decided to adopt a similar two-man forward-facing configuration as standard for the flight deck of its new 767 airliner, and began modifying aircraft already completed.

Indonesia is not the only corner of the Third World that is exerting a major influence on aviation today. One of the most remarkable recent stories of success in aircraft manufacture by a new company is that of Embraer of Brazil. Under the leadership of a small team of talented men, including chairman/chief executive Ozires Silva and technical director Guido Pessotti,

this twelve-year-old company has become one of the top ten manufacturers outside the Soviet Union in terms of numbers of aircraft built annually. More significantly, it has sold large quantities of its best known product, the 21-passenger Bandeirante twin-turboprop transport, in the USA, the birthplace of commuter air travel.

By the spring of 1982 the 400th Bandeirante was on the final assembly line in the Embraer works at São José dos Campos, São Paulo State. Eighty per cent of those built in 1981 were exported, with nearly half of all exports over a three-year period going to 21 US operators. One of them, Dolphin Airways, notched up the Bandeirante's one millionth flight hour in early 1982. Further south, a ten-year-old boy became the 100,000th patient transported in one of the Bandeirante air ambulances flown by the Mexican Institute of Social Security (IMSS) when he was carried from his home town of Los Mochis, Sinaloa, to Guadalajara for lung surgery. By then IMSS had flown their Brazilian ambulances a total of 2.5 million miles, though the young patient was more impressed by the fact that a woman pilot was at the controls.

Bandeirante air ambulance of IMSS of Mexico. *(Embraer)*

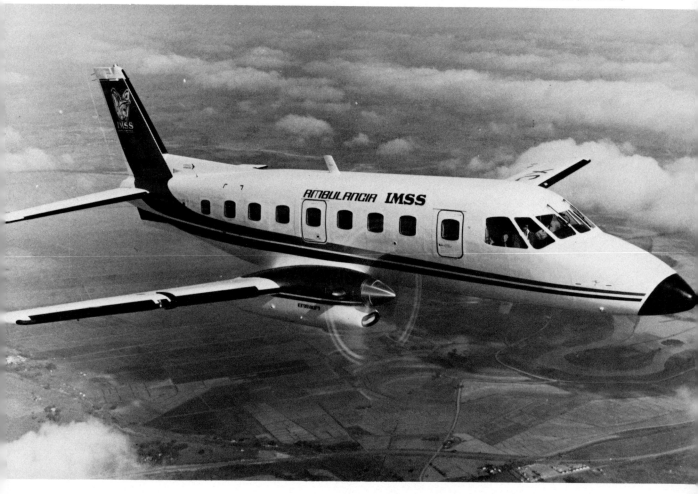

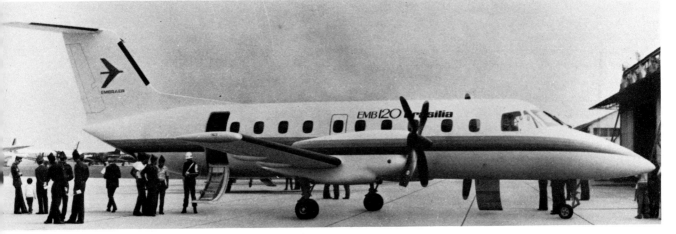

Mock-up of the 30-passenger Brasilia, under development by Embraer as the next step beyond the successful Bandeirante programme. *(Embraer)*

A young British pilot whose name appears frequently among the photo credits in *Jane's All the World's Aircraft* has spent much of his professional life flying Datapost mail by night between cities in the UK and to the Continent on behalf of the Post Office. Just before the *Review* went to press he qualified to fly a Bandeirante instead of the Cessna Titan he had flown previously. His verdict of "a thoroughly honest and uncomplicated aircraft" is shared by a huge number of pilots internationally, and this must augur well for the Bandeirante's big brother, the 30-passenger Brasilia, which is due to fly for the first time in 1983. Covering an area four-fifths the size of Europe, both east and west, and with poor surface communications, Brazil has a requirement for domestic air services comparable with that of Indonesia.

As well as its transports, Embraer also produces combat types, in partnership with Italy. The manufacture of 182 AT-26 Xavante (Aermacchi MB.326GB) attack/trainers is being followed by joint development with Aeritalia and Aermacchi of a potent little single-seat jet known as the AM-X, capable of performing interdiction, anti-ship, reconnaissance and close support duties. Its likely capability is emphasised by the fact that it will replace the G.91, G.91Y, F-104G and

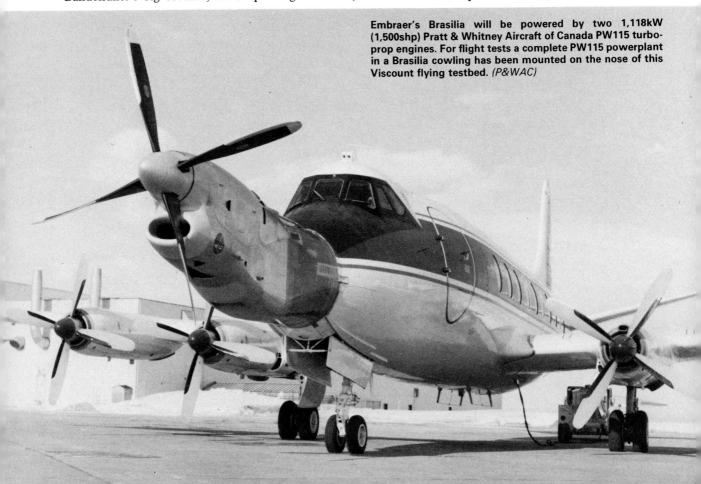

Embraer's Brasilia will be powered by two 1,118kW (1,500shp) Pratt & Whitney Aircraft of Canada PW115 turboprop engines. For flight tests a complete PW115 powerplant in a Brasilia cowling has been mounted on the nose of this Viscount flying testbed. *(P&WAC)*

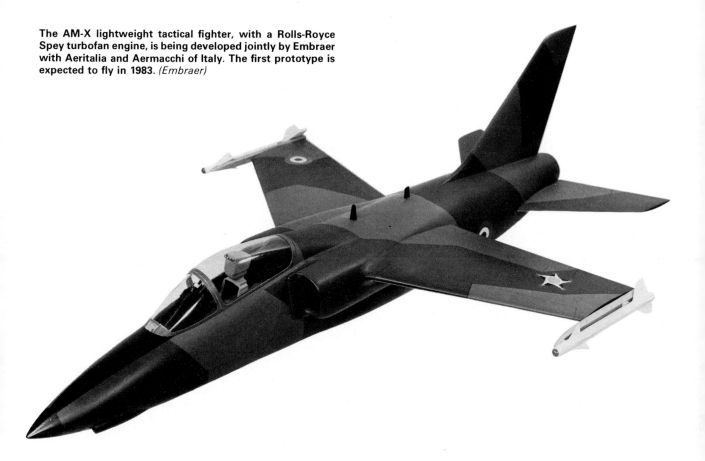

The AM-X lightweight tactical fighter, with a Rolls-Royce Spey turbofan engine, is being developed jointly by Embraer with Aeritalia and Aermacchi of Italy. The first prototype is expected to fly in 1983. (Embraer)

F-104S Starfighter in Nato service with Italian Air Force squadrons in Europe. It will in fact be a junior companion of the Tornado, currently one of the world's most formidable combat aircraft.

A more modest close support aircraft that has been in the news in 1982, as a result of the conflict in the Falkland Islands, is the twin-turboprop Pucará, built by Brazil's neighbour, Argentina. Troops subjected to its low-level attacks in the opening stages of the campaign found it "a nasty little beast". Its manoeuvrability and capacity to operate from short, rough airstrips, carrying a variety of weapons, suggested that the larger, faster and far more heavily armed American A-10 Thunderbolt II, designed for similar duties in front-line areas, might be a formidable weapon on Nato's central front in Europe. But the lessons of the Falkland Islands must be studied with care.

Jane's All the World's Aircraft has to be international and non-political. For that reason an article of this kind, by its editor, must concentrate on strategy, tactics and hardware without commenting on the political or moral aspects of any military campaign. The first clear lesson of the Falklands operation is one that it had in common with the Korean War. There, more than 30 years ago, the US Air Force fought the first jet-to-jet engagements against the new Soviet MiG-15 fighter. The Americans' ability to protect themselves was reduced by the fact that the MiGs, flown by Chinese

pilots, could escape by dashing back over the Yalu River to regain their bases in China, where US fighter pilots were forbidden to follow. This prompted the post-Korea view that no air force should ever again be trapped into a situation in which it and its friends could be attacked freely by aircraft operating from bases that for political reasons were secure from counter-attack. Yet the Royal Air Force and Royal Navy pilots in the Falklands found themselves fighting in precisely similar circumstances, with one hand tied behind their backs.

While Argentinian pilots could fly over the Falklands and surrounding waters to attack and sink Royal Navy ships, the bases from which they operated on the Argentinian mainland were declared to be prohibited targets.

The weapon used with greatest effect by the Argentinian air forces was the French Exocet air-to-surface missile, with which a number of British ships were sunk. Its accuracy and effectiveness should have surprised no-one. The Argentinian Navy was known to have received some of the 14 Super Etendard fighters that it had ordered from Dassault in 1979, and these aircraft were known to be able to carry Exocet. As long ago as 1969 the foreword to *Jane's All the World's Aircraft* had commented: "Exocet ... is designed to race towards its target at high subsonic speed, in all weathers, a mere six to ten feet above the water, over a

39

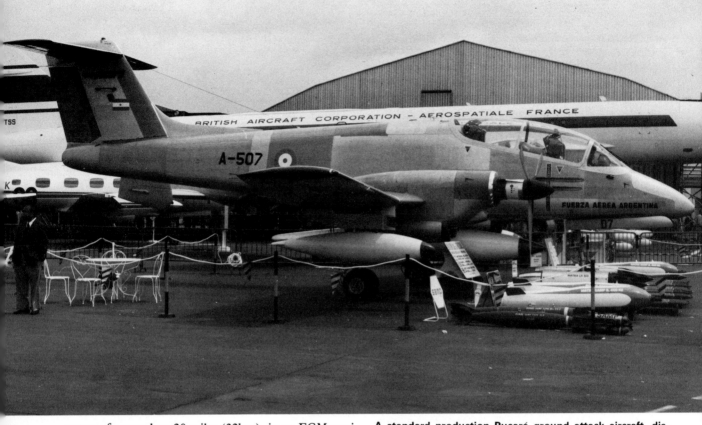

A standard production Pucará ground attack aircraft, displayed with some of the weapons it can carry, at the Paris Air Show. *(Austin J. Brown)*

range of more than 20 miles (32km), in an ECM environment. How can one possibly defend a ship against such a missile?''

One answer, of course, is to ensure that the carrier aircraft is detected before it comes close enough to launch its missile. Back in 1921-23, off America, General ''Billy'' Mitchell demonstrated how easily undefended battleships could be sunk by air attack, and was subsequently court-martialled for insubordination. In

December 1941 the two most powerful ships of the British Far Eastern Fleet, HMS *Prince of Wales* and HMS *Repulse*, were sent to the bottom by Japanese torpedo-bombers when they ventured beyond the range of RAF air cover. After decades of such lessons, in 1982 nobody should have despatched naval forces into an area where they could be subjected to Exocet missile attack without the protection offered by early-

RAF Harrier GR3, fitted with 2in rocket pods, photographed before its departure for combat operations around the Falkland Islands. *(RAF)*

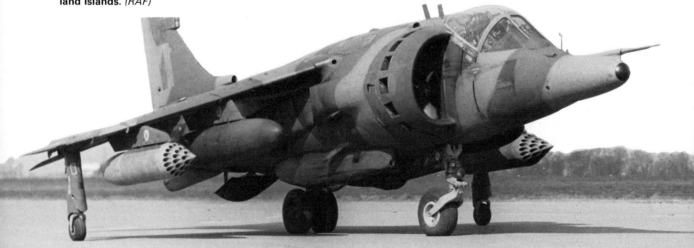

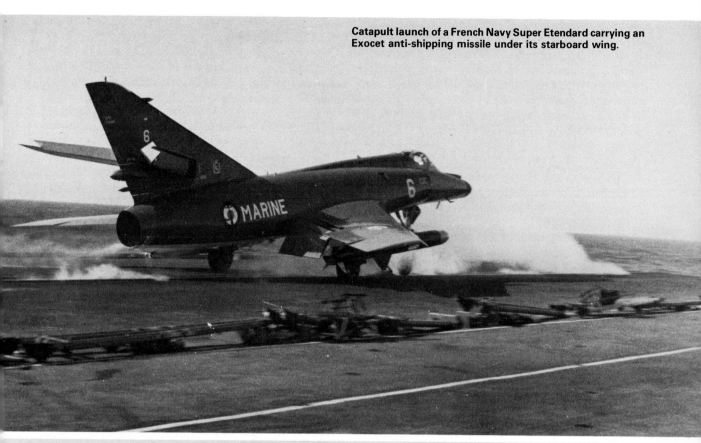

Catapult launch of a French Navy Super Etendard carrying an Exocet anti-shipping missile under its starboard wing.

This LRV-2 research RPV is being used by Nasa for the first stage in a programme that may lead eventually to advanced aircraft able to orbit at a height of 100,000ft for periods of several days. Such aircraft, referred to as "poor man's satellites," could be made of plastics and equipped for early-warning radar duties, taking over this role from the manned and more vulnerable E-3A Sentry.

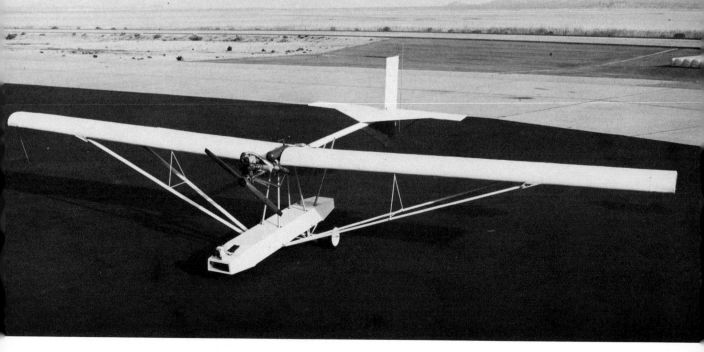

warning aircraft. Unfortunately, the last Royal Navy Gannets equipped for such a task were scrapped long ago for economic reasons, and not replaced by any type able to give cover to the Fleet in waters so far from home. The ships that tried to fill the gap by acting as radar pickets paid the price.

This is only one lesson of the Falklands campaign that should never be forgotten. There are others worthy of study:

* The only aircraft that can be guaranteed to continue flying in a front-line combat area are those which are independent of airfields, like the British V/Stol Harriers and helicopters.
* The value of heavy-lift helicopters to move stores around base areas at home, between shore and ship, and in combat areas cannot be overstated.
* Aircraft have limited hope of survival at any height against well manned surface-to-air missile defences.
* Because of its unique manoeuvrability the Harrier has proved itself as effective in an air-to-air role as its protagonists have claimed.
* The odds are still against pilots, however brave and however good their aircraft, if they have to fly a long distance to a combat zone and then engage in combat.
* An aircraft industry competent enough to develop and fit flight-refuelling equipment to transport and maritime reconnaissance aircraft, and air-launched missiles and new-type rocket pods to types as diverse as the Harrier GR3 and Nimrod, in a few weeks and then send the aircraft confidently into action is an asset that few nations possess, or deserve after years of penny-pinching on defence.

The most depressing feature of this war that ought never to have happened is that the politicians of both sides are unlikely to have learned all the lessons that it should have taught. The clearest lesson of all, at a time when the UK is preparing to spend £11,000 million on Trident submarine-launched missile systems, is that the Royal Navy's current possession of Polaris submarines did not deter Argentina from occupying the Falkland Islands. Nor were such missiles of the slightest use in the subsequent campaign. For half the cost of the Trident programme Britain could buy squadrons of B-1B strategic bombers able to play a major deterrent/attack role in any conceivable kind of military confrontation, nuclear or conventional, independently or as a component of Nato. A nation equipped primarily to confront with submarine-launched missiles a superpower that could remove its territory and people from the map within minutes of the outbreak of hostilities, but which lacks key weapons for limited campaigns, is in a very unhappy position in the world of the 1980s.

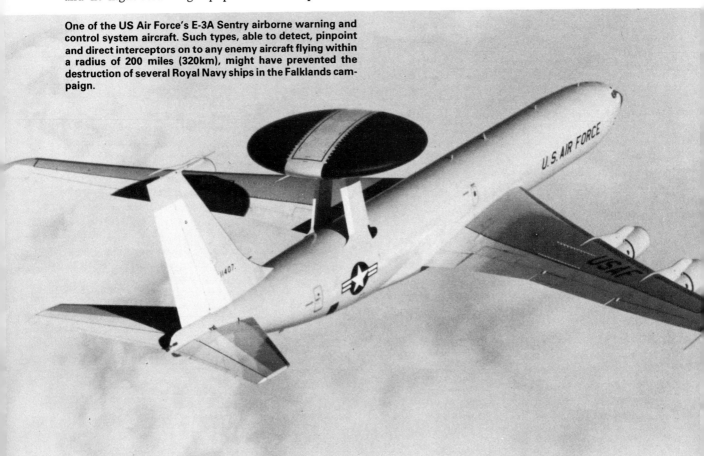

One of the US Air Force's E-3A Sentry airborne warning and control system aircraft. Such types, able to detect, pinpoint and direct interceptors on to any enemy aircraft flying within a radius of 200 miles (320km), might have prevented the destruction of several Royal Navy ships in the Falklands campaign.

Strange Wings, Strange Things

DON DOWNIE

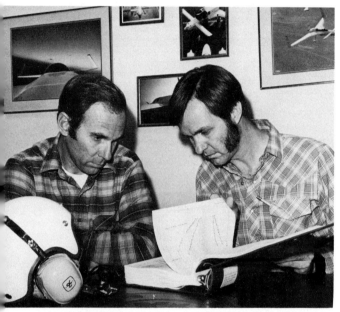

Burt Rutan (right) studying Fairchild Republic NGT data. (Downie and Associates)

There's a civilian flight-test centre in the southern California desert, midway between the US Air Force/Nasa test base at Edwards Dry Lake and the US Navy Weapons Centre at China Lake. This site, located beside broad runways dating back to the Second World War, is in a sparsely populated area where the risks of primary flight testing are acceptable.

It is from the hangars and ramps at Mojave, California, that some of the most advanced designs in private and commercial aviation have first flown. Many of these strange wings came from the prolific drawing board of Burt Rutan, who has introduced a whole new approach to lightplane design and construction. Almost all Rutan's designs are of a canard configuration, with the smaller lifting surface at the front of the airframe and the main wings aft. Composite construction is used throughout.

Rutan is already known throughout the world as the designer of the pace-setting little VariEze, second after the VariViggen in a line of fuel-efficient, high-performance two-seat homebuilts. This tiny white aeroplane began as a 181kg (399lb) empty weight pro-

totype with a 47kW (63hp) Volkswagen engine, but the design was promptly enlarged to produce a second prototype with a 254kg (560lb) empty weight and a 67kW (90hp) Continental O-200 engine. More than 400 of these homebuilts are now flying throughout the world, with a number in England, France, Switzerland and Australia, while about 1,600 others are under construction. Don Foreman of Hextable, Kent, England, flying G-LASS, captured several point-to-point class world records with his VariEze, including a flight from Malta to England.

Thousands of plans sold

More than 3,500 sets of VariEze plans were sold between 1976 and the introduction of the larger Long-EZ late in 1979, while by 1982 the success of the Long-EZ had itself resulted in the delivery of more than 2,000

Rutan VariEze.

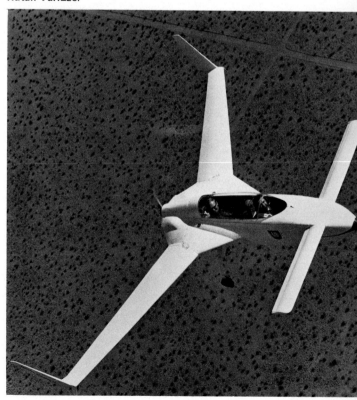

43

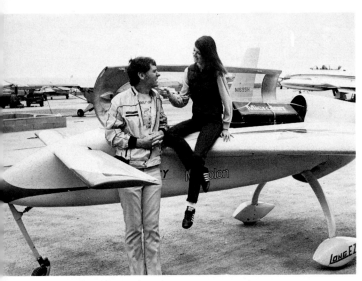

sets of plans to amateur constructors. A high percentage of these sales have resulted in aircraft under construction. At last count 16 of the larger model (Long-EZ) had actually flown, and eight world records had been gained by the aircraft built by Burt's brother Dick. A non-stop, non-refuelled flight from Anchorage, Alaska, to Grand Turk Island, West Indies, on June 5/6, 1981, set an impressive straight-line record in FAI Class C-1-b of 7,344.56km (4,563.7 miles) in a flying time of 30hr 8min. The modified Long-EZ has a larger, 119kW (160hp), Avco Lycoming O-320 engine for air show demonstrations and a 556lit (147 US gal) fuel capacity, and burned 4.71gal/hr on the record flight. More recently, this same Long-EZ has set Class C-1-b speed records for aircraft under 1,000kg over distances of 500km, 1,000km and 2,000km. Dick Rutan managed 340.55km/hr (211.61mph) and 334.49km/hr (207.84mph) for the 500km and 1,000km courses respectively, while Jeana Yeager was clocked at 329.24km/hr (204.58mph) for the 2,000km. The 2,000km dash required full throttle at low altitude for a distance equal to Los Angeles-Dallas. When this

Dick Rutan and Jeana Yeager with the record-breaking Long-EZ. *(Downie and Associates)*

Rutan Grizzly with (left to right) a VariViggen, two Long-EZs with nosewheels retracted, the Defiant and the Amsoil Racer. *(Downie and Associates)*

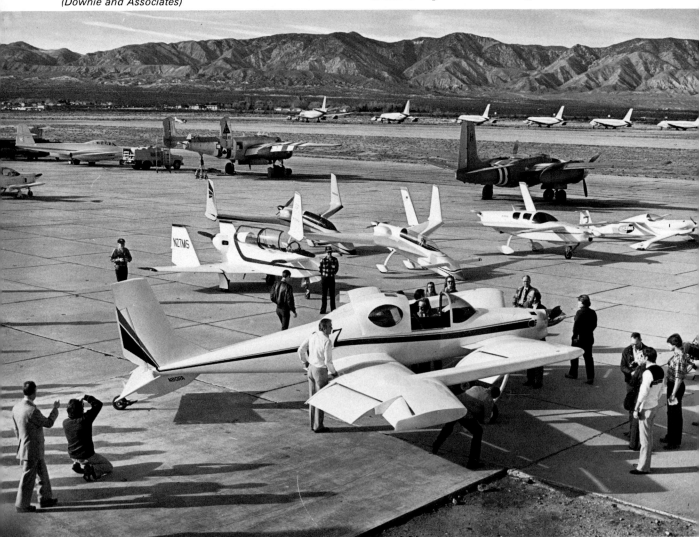

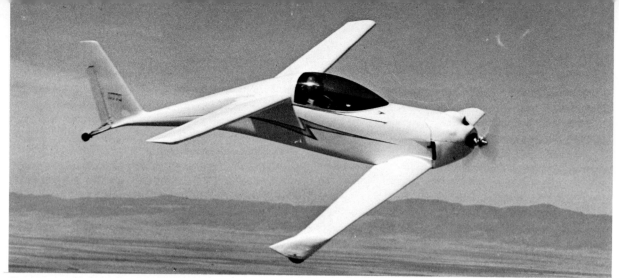

Quickie Aircraft Corporation Quickie. *(Downie and Associates)*

Long-EZ is clean it has a true airspeed of 359km/hr (223mph), dropping to 341km/hr (212mph) when the wing surfaces are spattered with insects.

A feature of the VariEze and Long-EZ that has added further to the aircrafts' unusual appearance on the ground is the fact that the nosewheel and glassfibre strut must be retracted before the pilot leaves the cockpit. If the pilot climbs out of the cockpit with the nose gear extended, the tail drops, damaging both winglets and propeller. If the nose was ballasted to eliminate this peculiarity, the added weight would result in very long take-off rolls and make the aircraft extremely difficult to handle on the ground.

The Thoughts of "Reverend Rutan"

Some irreverent visitors to Rutan's regular weekly open house each Saturday from 10 a.m., with flight demonstrations at noon, comment that these mini-seminars are just like going to church with the "Reverend Rutan" in the pulpit. These same people suggest that when an Eze is parked nose-down, it should be pointed toward Mojave.

Burt Rutan's list of flying credentials is long and varied. His first homebuilt design, the VariViggen, was begun near Mojave in 1968 when Burt was employed as a civilian test engineer by the US Air Force at Edwards Air Force Base. The VariViggen, influenced to some degree by Sweden's successful canard fighter, the Saab JA37 Viggen, was completed and test-flown in Newton, Kansas, while Rutan was project engineer on the Bede BD-5 project.

The tiny banana-shaped Quickie came from Rutan's drawing board but was really the brainchild of Gene Sheehan and Tom Jewett (killed this year while test-flying the *Free Enterprise* record-attempt aircraft), two Californian development engineers who had searched for four years to find a suitable low-cost engine for a sports plane. After they had selected the 13.5kW (18hp) Onan two-cylinder, four-stroke, direct-drive engine, Burt Rutan was commissioned to develop the airframe. The result was another novel planform, with the main landing wheels in the tips of the canard. After three months of design and prototype construction Rutan completed his contract and went on to other projects. Sheehan is now successfully marketing the Quickie and the follow-on side-by-side two-seat Q2.

One of the most promising Rutan designs since the VariEze is the twin-engined, push-pull Defiant. Developed as a proof-of-concept one-off, the spacious five-seater will cruise 1,931km (1,200 miles) at 354km/hr (220mph) and 12gal/hr on the power of its twin 134kW (180hp) Avco Lycoming engines. The prototype has logged more than 600hr, including uneventful trips to Alaska and Mexico. Rutan has hopes of flying this aircraft to Hawaii and eventually to Europe. Despite a number of promising offers, the only follow-on effort is a second aircraft now being built in Alaska by VariEze prizewinner Fred Keller, who won the coveted EAA Builder's Award at the Oshkosh annual fly-in and show. Keller is currently building a cleaned-up version of the prototype Defiant, with a canopy change and, possibly, constant-speed propellers.

Rutan keeps control

Rutan's reluctance to modify the Defiant for production results from several financing proposals that would have robbed the designer of effective control over the finished product. Rutan also feels that the Defiant is too complex a project for most homebuilders and is therefore not trying to market plans. However, it is too soon to write off the Defiant. All that have flown it, myself included, agree that the Defiant is far too fine a flying machine to remain a singleton.

One builder's effort to emulate the Defiant concept has resulted in the Gemini, developed in nearby San Diego, California. This variation, a side-by-side two-seat push-pull aeroplane powered by two Volkswagen modified car engines, made its debut at Oshkosh in August 1982.

Rutan's rare birds come in all shapes and sizes. Take the Predator, a huge turboprop-powered agricultural aircraft designed as a feasibility study for an indepen-

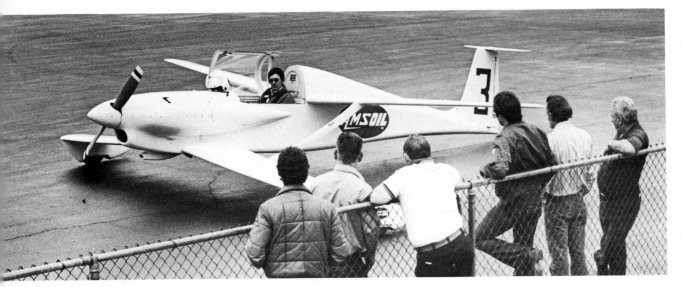

Mortensen/Rutan Amsoil Racer. *(Downie and Associates)*

Grizzly in flight over Mojave. *(Downie and Associates)*

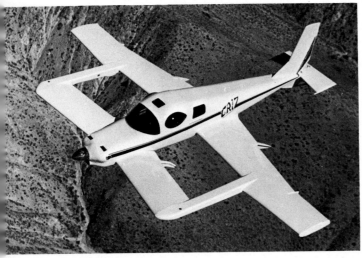

dent contractor. To date there is no prototype, but the specification calls for a 3,039kg (6,700lb) payload of insecticide to be dispersed over a swath width 58 per cent greater than that offered by existing agricultural aircraft. The pilot would sit in the leading edge of the fin, while the wings extend fore and aft in what is almost a diamond pattern. This study may well result in a production aeroplane, as the original contractor is even now seeking finance for a full-scale testbed.

Former FAA air traffic controller Dan Mortensen competes in biplane air races. After several seasons of flying a Mong racer and viewing other exhaust stacks ahead of him at the finish line, he asked Rutan to design a completely new biplane racer to beat all existing competition. Rutan produced the design and Mortensen, aided by two EAA chapters in the Sacramento, California, area, built the biplane. During its first outing in Reno, the Amsoil Racer (named after Mortensen's sponsor) finished third in the biplane class, even

allowing for penalties for cutting two pylons. More recently this Rutan design established an unofficial three-kilometre course record of 377.58km/hr (234.62mph) for the small C-1-b class. This was achieved in spite of the fact that the 119kW (160hp) Avco Lycoming IO-320 engine was running rough and had a compression of 40:80 on one cylinder. This aircraft looked well set to win at Reno 1982 and could break several class records. (See also *New Aircraft of the Year*, page 87.)

Handling the Defiant and VariEze

As an aviation reporter living in southern California, I have had more than a casual acquaintance with Rutan's engineering efforts. I flew with him when the Defiant had 30hr to its credit and found the aircraft stable, forgiving and free of the many paste-pot-and-gun-tape shortcomings so frequently found in a new prototype. Later I flew in the VariEze and was checked out by Dick Rutan for a solo flight in the prototype Long-EZ. The latter is a magnificent machine with docile handling, low approach speed and a consistent 298km/hr (185mph) cruising speed on the power of its 85.75kW (115hp) Avco Lycoming O-235 engine.

More recently I was privileged to fly the single-seat Amsoil Racer. Though this competition aircraft is only 6.10m (20ft) long, with a span of 6.71m (22ft), the cockpit is surprisingly comfortable. The side-stick control used in all the designs mentioned so far takes little getting used to: you just hold the neat little control column with your fingertips and enjoy the flying. Checking out in a single-seater is done best at big, quiet, isolated strips like Mojave, where there was 2,925m (9,600ft) of good hard runway for my initial landing in the racer. As it was, I used almost half of the available strip.

The strange-winged Grizzly

Next in the chronology of the RAF (Rutan Aircraft

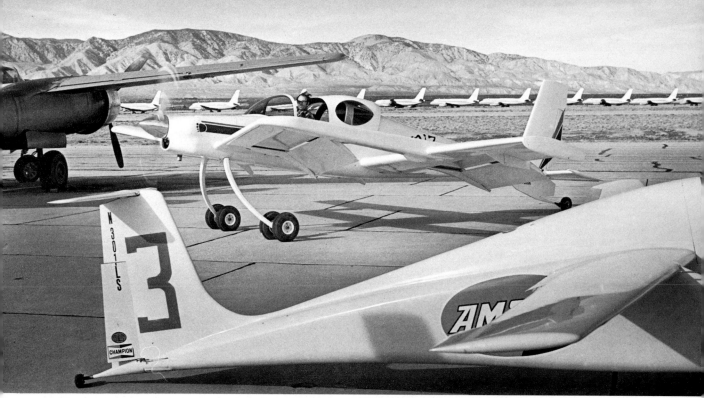

Grizzly taxis past the Amsoil Racer, with mothballed Boeing
707s in the background. *(Downie and Associates)*

Factory) is another design that Burt developed to prove
that canard designs would fly slowly as well as rapidly.
His Model 77 (originally conceived in 1977) is called
the Grizzly and was first presented to the aviation press
early in 1982. The Grizzly looks like nothing ever seen
in flight before and is truly one of Mojave's strange-
winged things.

The Grizzly is the result of a visit to Alaska by Rutan
in the Defiant. He looked at some of the bush aircraft
and went back to Mojave to produce the Grizzly, a
proof-of-concept research aircraft with four large
Fowler flaps that increase the wing area by 60 per cent.
It has a rugged landing gear with two pairs of low-
pressure tyres for off-field landings, and a fold-down
back seat for level-attitude camping for two people;
amphibious floats are being studied.

Recently I joined the designer on a brief demonstration flight. The wind was gusting 20kt, as it does much
of the time at Mojave, so Rutan (a very good pilot for an
aeronautical engineer) cranked down half flaps and we
took off across the runway and into the wind. We
pulled up over the tower and then the designer took a
minute or two to relax as we wound our way between
the high fins of old Boeing 707s, long since retired from
airline service and parked in dry desert storage along
one runway at Mojave at $50 per month per aircraft.
Rutan had a grin on his bewhiskered face as the Grizzly
made smooth S-turns around the tail feathers of these
once-proud birds. "This is fun," he said casually. We
landed across the runway with a ground roll of perhaps
30m (100ft).

A whole new research and development trend is
resulting from Rutan's efforts to design and build a
0.62-scale model of Fairchild Republic's NGT (Next
Generation Trainer) proposal for the USAF. Rutan
designed the structure and systems for this pint-sized
single-seater, which will ultimately grow into a full-size
side-by-side two-seat trainer prototype. In just eight
weeks Rutan and his crew went through a complete
flight-test programme and supplied the necessary
detailed engineering data for a 220-page report to back
up the full-scale effort.

Since that time a new company has been formed to
exploit this type of research and development, whereby
a design is fabricated to a smaller scale from a mouldless
composite sandwich of unidirectional carbon fibre and
glassfibre.

The self-launching Solitaire

The very latest design from Rutan's team is a single-
seat self-launching sailplane for recreational flying.
The prototype will be entered in a new design competition sponsored by the Soaring Society of America and
Western Flyer magazine, based in Tacoma, Washington. There are a number of national and international
entries in this contest. Called Solitaire, the new powered sailplane has a fixed internal engine (currently a
12.7kW; 17hp Cuyuna, used in many microlights) and
a fully retractable propeller. Basically a 12.5m sailplane, Solitaire will be marketed in the same way as the
Long-EZ, with Rutan supplying the plans and
approved vendors offering materials and many hard-
to-construct assemblies. For example, the entire composite fuselage of Solitaire will be available from a
nearby shop, cutting down appreciably on the construction time.

Solitaire is a true sailplane, not a microlight. Rutan expects builders to run the engine for not more than 10min at a time, just long enough to get to height and soar. "From there on, the spoilers will serve as a throttle in good soaring conditions," explains the designer.

The British 18.6kW (25hp) Garrett two-cylinder engine weighing only 7.3kg (16lb) will also be tried out in Solitaire. "We have several options in powerplants," says Rutan. "The Cuyuna people have excellent product support, so we'll see about a permanent engine after we get the aerodynamics cleaned up. We're after a 30:1 glide."

There remains one machine in this Rutan line of unusual aircraft that is hard to catalogue. It all began when RAF submitted an unsolicited proposal to Nasa for a feasibility study of an adjustable skew-wing aircraft. The design came from Rutan, with the Ames Industrial Corporation actually building the jet-powered test vehicle. Called the AD-1, the skew-wing aircraft has completed a flight programme at nearby Edwards Air Force Base. The wing slews 60° at the pilot's command, making this the world's first manned adjustable skew-wing aircraft.

Round-the-world record attempt

At the beginning of 1982 at least two companies were looking at the possibility of tackling what would be a unique feat: a flight around the world, non-stop, non-refuelled. Between December 5 and 8, 1981, Jerry Mullens flew the Javelin-prepared Phoenix single-handed over a distance of 16,206km (10,070 miles) in a flying time of 73hr 2min. This flight proved not only the longest in terms of duration and distance ever achieved by an unrefuelled aircraft crewed by a pilot only, but showed that an unrefuelled round-the-world flight was undoubtedly possible by an aircraft not produced by one of the world's major aircraft manufactur-

Below Rutan's 0·62-scale version of the Fairchild Republic NGT trainer. *(Rutan)*

Bottom Rutan Solitaire self-launching sailplane under construction in the workshop, with the scale version of the NGT trainer hanging from the ceiling. *(Downie and Associates)*

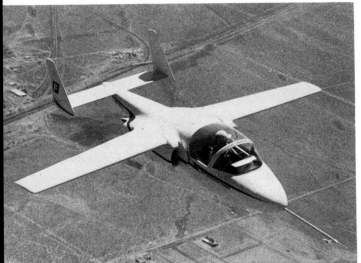

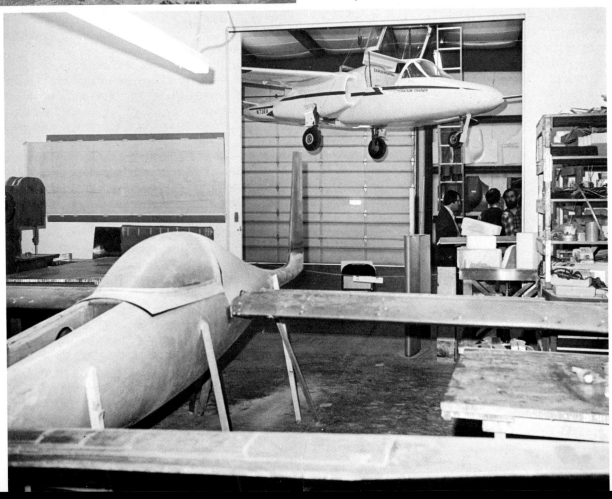

ers. The Quickie team of Sheehan and Jewett, located just east on the ramp at Mojave, were relying on their *Free Enterprise* (formerly Big Bird), an overgrown sailplane with a turbocharged 100.5kW (135hp) PZL-F4A-235, when tragedy intervened in July 1982 (see page 101).

Down the flight line at Rutan's end of the field, Dick Rutan and his partner, Jeana Yeager (no relation to Chuck Yeager), have formed Voyager Aircraft. Their business card reads: "Round the World ★ Non-stop ★ Non-refuelled Flight." Talk with Dick Rutan about his proposal and he doesn't say very much: "Just as soon as we have an adequate sponsor, we'll give out the details. We already have the press releases written. Before that time, there's nothing to say. If we can't get adequate financing, there just won't be a record attempt and we won't have to back down from some outlandish statements that had been made."

However, much has already been written about Voyager, most of it bootlegged from proposals submitted to potential sponsors. It is likely that Voyager would be a huge canard push-pull with two differently rated Avco Lycoming engines. The fuselage would have side windows, with nothing for forward visibility except a small bubble over the pilot's compartment. Fuel would be carried in just about every part of the airframe, including the portion of the cabin where the second pilot in the two-person crew could sleep during the estimated ten days' flight time. This sleeping area has been designed to start out as a collapsible fuel cell that will flatten out once that portion of the fuel is burned off, a system pioneered on Dick Rutan's record Long-EZ flight from Alaska to the Caribbean. Jeana made the flight from Mojave to Anchorage in the back seat of the Long-EZ with an empty water bed for a cushion. At the take-off point the water bed was filled with fuel and Jeana took an airliner to Florida.

An artist's impression based on bootlegged information showed a huge canard with a wing span of 30m (100ft) or more and a length of 7.6m (25ft). Speed was quoted as 177km/hr (110mph). Burt Rutan has had a quiet laugh at the drawing, which appeared in a British newspaper. The sketch had been modified to eliminate the forward canard and replace it with a conventional elevator-stabiliser. "I guess that the artist just didn't believe that we really meant to put the canard up front, but we do!" comments Rutan.

There are a number of rumours about the Voyager project, but some things seem certain. It is likely that the design is nearly finalised and that some construction has already begun; one of the main attributes of Rutan's composite structures is the fact that they can be built quickly with a minimum of tooling. While Sheehan and Jewett's *Free Enterprise* was to take off from a dolly and land on the bottom of the fuselage, Rutan may be considering a two-piece landing gear, part of which would be dropped after the heavyweight

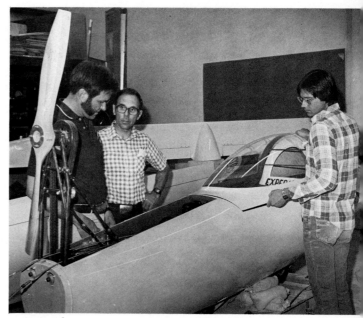

Burt Rutan inspects the propeller drive system of the Solitaire self-launching sailplane. *(Downie and Associates)*

take-off, with the remainder used for landing. Rutan believes that he can save more weight by not strengthening the bottom of the fuselage and carrying a portion of the landing gear.

One take-off method might call for a tow from a car or truck during the initial portion of the take-off roll. If the home base at Mojave, California, is used, there is a 9,600ft main runway with nothing but miles of low sagebrush off the end. If that isn't long enough, the 24km (15 miles) of dry lake bed at Edwards Air Force Base, used for Space Shuttle Orbiter landings, is less than 48km (30 miles) from Rutan's factory.

The second engine on the Voyager need operate only for the first two days of the flight until some of the fuel load is burned off. Then the propeller could be feathered and the engine could serve as insurance against problems with the continuously running rear-mounted unit.

What next?
What's new from Rutan's Aircraft Factory? They have bid for and hope to win the contract to build a life-sized flyable model of Chuck Yeager's X-1. The model is to be flown underneath the B-29 operated by the Confederate Air Force. The X-1 model will be used for a new film centred on Tom Wolfe's best-selling novel *The Right Stuff*. Under present plans the X-1 model will not actually be dropped, so it has only to be stressed to fly at slightly under 320km/hr (200mph) in the bay of the B-29. A previous model built by a Hollywood model-builder proved to be unacceptable for flight scenes when the wings drooped markedly after being tested with weights on the ground. When the weights were removed, the droop remained, and there followed a rush call to Rutan's shop.

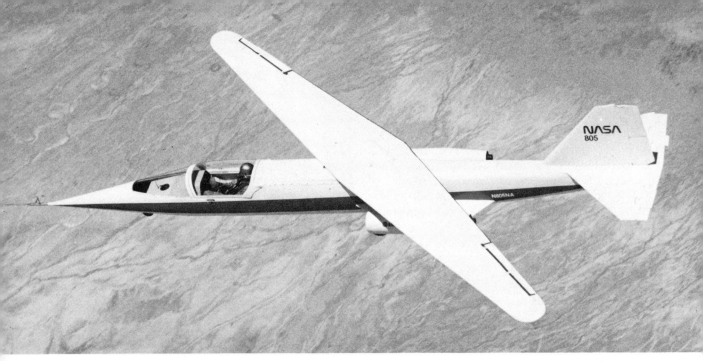

Rutan skew-wing aircraft, known to Nasa as the AD-1.

The X-1 project, while not an engineering challenge, would help finance Rutan's small shop, which employs six to eight people. If possible Rutan hopes to buy back the model and mount it outside his office, just as the Air Force has done with the real thing at nearby Edwards Air Force Base. However, Rutan would put the epoxy and carbon-fibre model to use, analysing the effects of the hot desert sun on the composite structure of the aircraft.

At the time of writing, Rutan has a wind-tunnel model of a canard 36-passenger commuter aircraft being tested by Nasa. If the money becomes available for a research project, he is prepared to build a scaled-down flying model to prove the basic design. Rutan believes it would take about $1 million to design and build a half-scale model. As for the worldwide expansion of microlight flying, Rutan will only say: "Beyond Solitaire, I can neither confirm nor deny rumours that we're developing an ultralight."

There is a great deal of cloak-and-dagger in this very competitive field of aircraft development. Rutan has recently rented three tiny office rooms in "downtown Mojave" (at 2,787 souls, population is the same as the altitude in feet). This hideaway enables Rutan to work on the drawing board, preparing design studies and technical reports away from the telephone and visitors.

A visit to Mojave is truly an adventure in strange wings and strange things. What can be seen here in the shrouded hangars, simple work areas and back rooms foreshadows what we may well see on tomorrow's production lines.

Quickie Aircraft Corporation *Free Enterprise* **flanked by a Quickie and Quickie Q2. The late Tom Jewett faces the camera.** *(Larry Willett)*

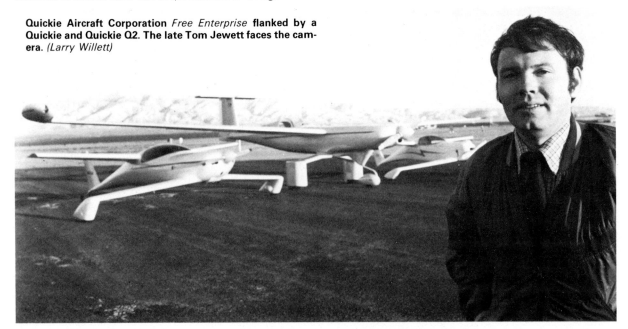

Bright Star 82

TERRY GANDER

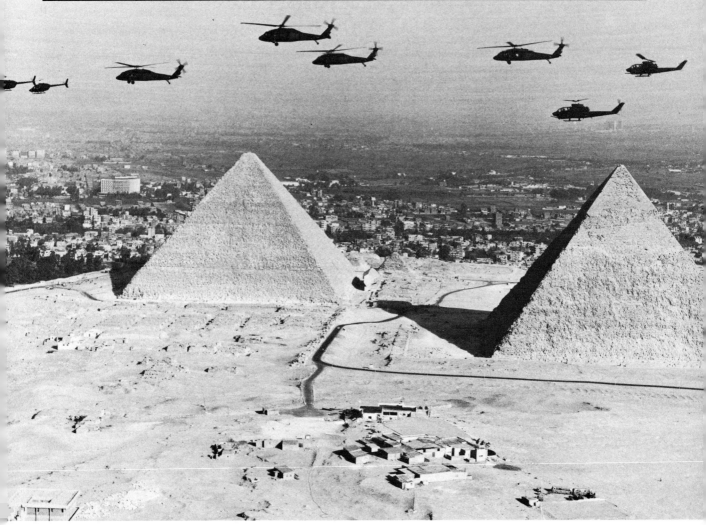

US Bell Kiowa, Sikorsky Black Hawk and AH-1S HueyCobra helicopters during the first Bright Star exercise. *(US Army)*

It is now generally acknowledged that the heady early days that followed the Camp David agreement have passed. One of the men that signed the agreement, Egyptian President Sadat, is dead. But even before his assassination it was clear that the spirit, if not the actual letter, of Camp David was as dead as its many Arab detractors wished it to be. One aspect of the agreement is however still very much in being, and that is the association between the United States and Egypt. The USA has voted huge sums in military and other aid to Egypt since Camp David, and in return has been offered facilities and other less tangible assistance in the Middle East. For the Americans this new source of co-operation and goodwill is very welcome, for one of the major current US military problems is that of forward support for America's Middle Eastern "fire brigade", the Rapid Deployment Force (RDF).

RDF was a child of the Kennedy administration, and of all recent US military innovations this one has come

51

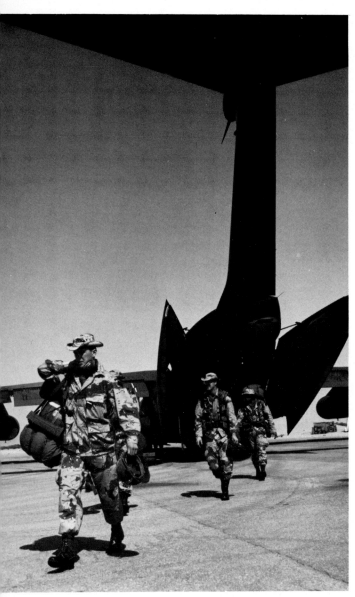

US forces begin arriving in Egypt for Bright Star 82.

RDF will not, by virtue of its very "fire-fighting" role, have time to cover long distances with the equipment it needs. The modern American fighting unit depends on a huge amount of heavy equipment of all kinds. This cannot be carried in suffiient quantity on normal US Air Force transport aircraft unless a great deal of time is allowed, and that is the one commodity that will be in short supply. Thus, even now, the Americans are setting up a chain of bases in the Middle East and Gulf regions where heavy equipment and supplies can be stockpiled ready for use. Much of this materiel is already loaded on supply ships, which are the only vehicles that can carry the amounts of heavy plant, weapons, AFVs, ammunition and other supplies that the modern US forces require. Most of these ships are currently based at Diego Garcia in the Indian Ocean, which is secure but still a long stretch from any potential flashpoint. There are very few other bases that meet these criteria of availability, location and security.

Close association with Egypt

This is where the close association with Egypt reveals its value. Nearby Israel is a very close ally of the USA but has made it plain that it can neither tolerate US forces in Israeli territory nor act as a supply base. Egypt will not act as a supply base either but is prepared to offer transit stations and is also willing to co-operate with military training and exercises in the area. The first example of this co-operation was seen when the first US-Egyptian Exercise Bright Star took place east of Cairo. Although it was a limited exercise, the Americans learned many unpleasant lessons. Infantry weapons became clogged with sand, helicopter blades eroded far too quickly, navigation across the desert tested both air and ground forces, and the extreme problems of maintenance in desert conditions revealed themselves.

The US forces have long carried out training in America's own desert areas, but it was discovered in Egypt that the firm going of California's Mojave Desert was very different from the soft blown sand of the Western Desert near Cairo. The fact that the Egyptian sand can get everywhere was one of the major lessons of the first Exercise Bright Star.

Planning for the second was well under way six months before the start date, November 14, 1981. Two combat battalions were to take part, and although the main action was set for Egypt, extra training was to take place in Oman, Somalia and the Sudan, all of which are seen as potential RDF staging and supply bases. Very soon it became clear that the combat forces would have a long support "tail". To back up the 2,000 or so combat troops, a further 2,000 support personnel were deemed necessary. Another 2,000 or so were needed for outside-Egypt operations, and suddenly Bright Star 82 was an expensive proposition. Many observers consider that a 1:1 ratio of back-up to combat personnel is

in for more than its fair share of criticism. The basic idea was, and still is, to provide the Pentagon with a flexible and rapid method of deploying a useful ground force in almost any part of the world. In practice this has meant the Persian Gulf from the very beginning. It was one thing to decree such a force, but it was quite another to set up, train and deploy it. The RDF has now been an established concept for nearly three years, but it is still incomplete, undermanned and understaffed. Most armies have such constraints imposed on them and get by, but for the Americans there is one basic problem that they cannot overcome without spending massive sums of money: the great distance between the United States and the theatre in which the RDF is likely to be deployed.

Distance alone can be overcome, as recently shown by the British Task Force in the South Atlantic, but the

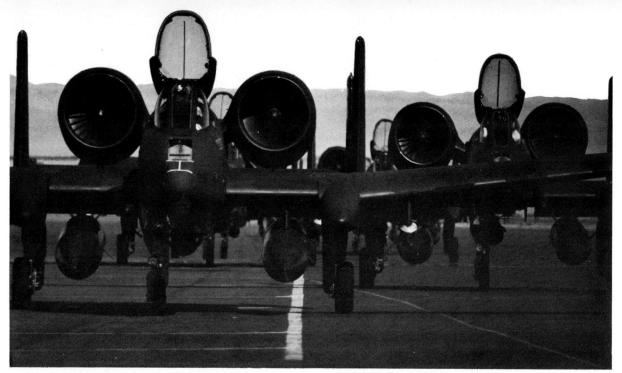

USAF Fairchild Republic A-10A Thunderbolt IIs of the 353rd Tactical Fighter Squadron prepare to attack enemy positions before the mass paratroop landings.

excessive, but that seems to be the way the US forces go to war these days. All manner of heavy equipment was deemed necessary from the very start, and even before the troops were being "warmed up" in extra training at their home bases the heavy equipment was on its way to Egypt from Savannah, Georgia.

Trucks, tanks and APCs
The heavy shipment comprised a total of 233 vehicles, mainly trucks, M113 APCs and M60 tanks. They were carried in a chartered West German roll-on, roll-off (ro-ro) ship, the MV *Cygnus*, which unloaded its cargo at Alexandria in readiness for the arrival of the 2nd Battalion, 21st Mechanised Infantry Regiment, 24th Mechanised Infantry Division. They had arrived in Egypt from November 4 by a variety of airborne methods, varying from chartered civil transports to C-141 StarLifters and C-5A Galaxies of Military Airlift

Command. With them came the host of US Air Force and Army personnel who would operate the supply, maintenance and personnel back-up facilities. Typical of these was an air-transportable hospital from Shaw Air Force Base, South Carolina, manned by the 354th Combat Support Group and carried in two MC-130 Hercules.

With the heavy equipment and full ground facilities at the ready — an unlikely event in a real war — the exercise proper got under way. November 14 saw a para-drop by the 2nd Battalion, 504th Infantry Landing Brigade, 82nd Airborne Division. Their way had been cleared the night before by an undisclosed number of men from the 5th Special Forces Group, normally based at Fort Bragg, Carolina (also the home base of the 82nd Airborne). They had been dropped silently from 10,000ft, using the long drop, low opening technique to avoid detection. Once on the ground

A USAF General Dynamics F-16A Fighting Falcon of the 388th Tactical Fighter Wing runs in to attack with low-drag bombs.

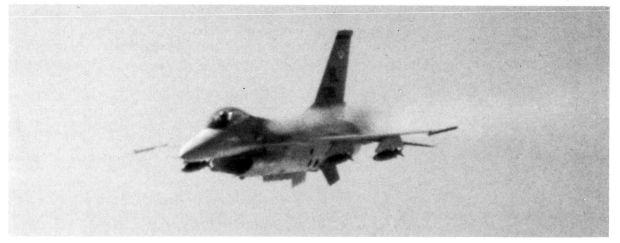

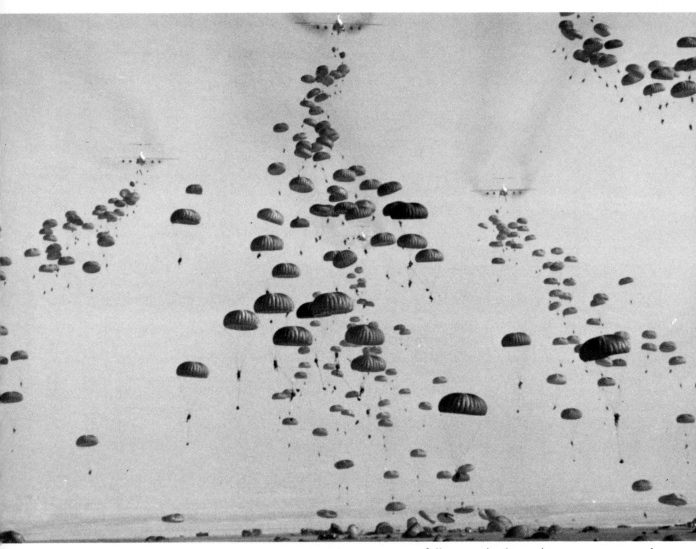

863 US and Egyptian paratroopers drop onto the Egyptian desert.

they set up a network of homing and marker beacons. Just before the main drop USAF A-10As and F-16s flew across the area to soften up possible enemy positions. The F-16s, from the 388th Tactical Fighter Wing, had flown in from their base at Hill AFB, Utah. (When this unit departed after the exercise it left four of its aircraft behind to provide training mounts for the Egyptian Air Force pilots who are to receive the F-16 this year.) The A-10As were from the 353rd Tactical Fighter Squadron at Myrtle Beach, Carolina.

Transatlantic paratroops

A total of 853 men from the 82nd Airborne and ten US-trained Egyptian paratroopers took part in the mass drop, which lasted six minutes from beginning to end. Creditable as this was, what was really remarkable was the fact that some aircraft had flown direct from South Carolina, while the others had broken their journey at European bases. The troops had been subjected

to a carefully contrived routine to overcome the debilitating effects of jet-lag and were comparatively fresh when they dropped in from six C-130s and 18 C-141s. Some of these aircraft also dropped heavy equipment on a total of 57 pallets. The troops were dropped from 245m (800ft) and the heavier loads from 460m (1,500ft). Compared with other similar efforts the drop was a great success: the only casualties were an officer with an injured hip and a "Gama Goat" truck that was crushed when its parachute failed to deploy.

From the start of the ground phase the theme was close co-operation with the Egyptian forces. Americans and Egyptians swapped and compared equipment and methods to their mutual benefit. Not all the comparisons went in favour of the Americans. It was painfully obvious to the US troops that the Egyptians preferred their Soviet-supplied AK-47 assault rifles to the American M-16. The early desert exercises had revealed that the M-16 was very vulnerable to sand contamination: if it was oiled it quickly clogged and jammed; if it was not oiled it jammed anyway. So the Americans had to clean their rifles at least three times every day, and fared no

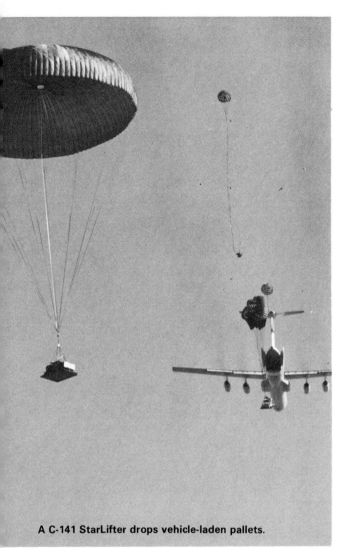

A C-141 StarLifter drops vehicle-laden pallets.

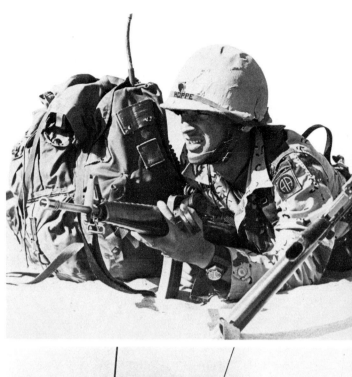

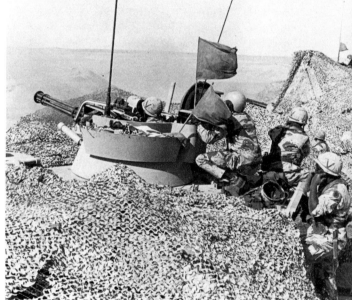

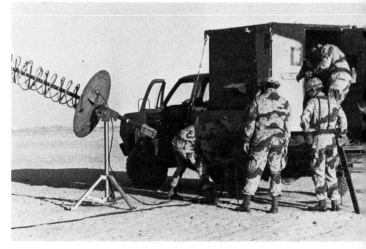

better with the M-60 machine gun. For the American troops it was a unique opportunity to sample Soviet weapons and equipment. There were live firings of SA-7 missiles and troops drove BTR-50PK APCs. The co-operation also extended to maintenance and back-up units. The maintenance men found themselves very much in close accord when performing most servicing tasks, although significant difficulties with language arose. Many US officers had undertaken crash courses in Arabic, but they could not be everywhere at once and translation problems often arose. The Egyptians, used to clear spoken English, had problems with American-accented Arabic, and it soon became clear that US Army language teaching still has some way to go before effective communications can be guaranteed.

Top **The sand caused major problems, jamming small arms and eroding helicopter blades.**

Middle **Land-mobile Vulcan M61A1 Gatling gun units in firing position.**

Right **A communications team from the Joint Communication Support Element (JCSE) was airlifted into the desert.**

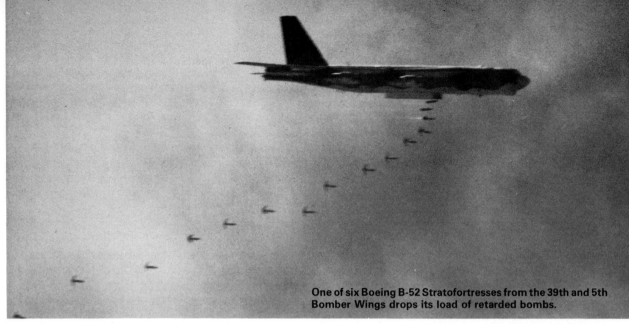

One of six Boeing B-52 Stratofortresses from the 39th and 5th Bomber Wings drops its load of retarded bombs.

On November 24 a spectacular firepower demonstration was carried out at Wadi Natroun, deep in the desert. As VIPs sipped their drinks under striped awnings, aircraft of both nations demonstrated their destructive capabilities in front of various foreign and other observers. The full show lasted 90min, the highlights being a bombing demonstration by six B-52s that had flown over from the US mainland. The aircraft came from the 39th and 5th Bomber Wings, based in North Dakota, and when they had dropped their loads of 500lb bombs they turned round and went straight home. The non-stop trip took almost 30 flying hours, and a small fleet of KC-135 tankers was used to keep the B-52s topped up. The crews must have been very tired at the end, but it was a very impressive demonstration of the long arm of American air power.

The Wadi Natroun demonstration also included Egyptian Air Force Tu-16 Badger bombers, MiG-17 Fresco and MiG-21 Fishbed fighters, Su-7 Fitter strike aircraft and French-built Mirage 5s. A combined helicopter assault was demonstrated by a mix of Soviet and Western-built aircraft (including a small number of Westland Commandos), while USAF pilots showed off the agility of the F-16 fire-control system and the low-level manoeuvrability of the A-10. A distant E-3A Sentry Awacs acted as master of ceremonies.

Away from Egypt, special units under the Bright Star 82 banner were working away in a quieter fashion. Special units of all kinds moved to Somalia, where they spent time working out how best to spend the military credits being extended to that country in exchange for base rights at several locations. A small logistics exercise was carried out at the port of Berbera, which is

The result of a B-52 run.

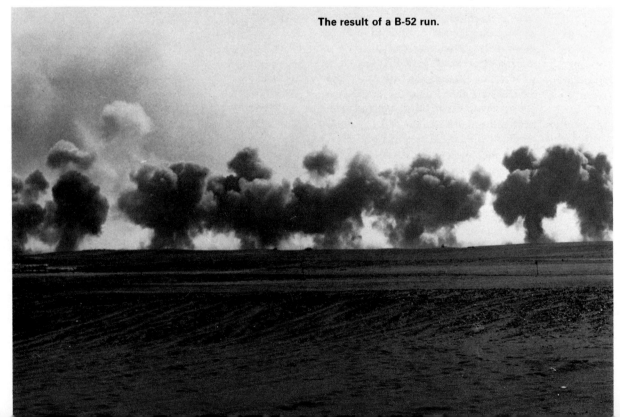

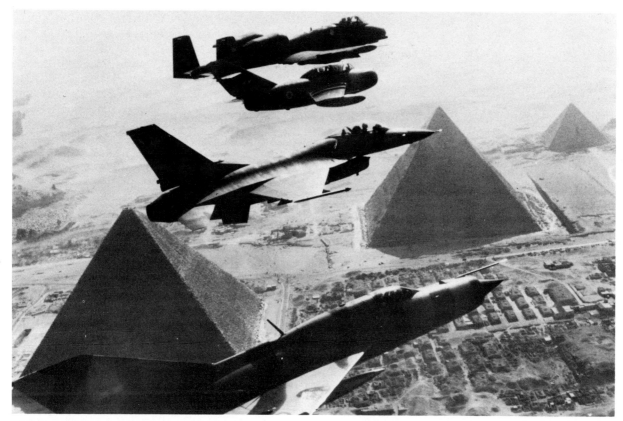

USAF A-10A and F-16A flying alongside Egyptian MiG-15UTI and MiG-21 over the pyramids of Giza.

being expanded with US financial aid to provide a deep-water harbour with nearby air landing facilities. In the Sudan 350 men from all three American services worked with the local armed forces for a period, again with local port and airfield access rights in mind.

Misgivings from the Gulf states

The largest outside-Egypt part of Bright Star 82 took place in Oman. The original plans for this Gulf state covered an amphibious landing by 1,800 US Marines, but things had changed by the time the landing actually took place. Several Gulf states were unhappy about the extent of American influence in their region, so by the time the big day arrived the planned landing had been much reduced in scale. At the Omanis' request, only 1,000 marines landed and the deepest beach-head penetration was only four miles, with the bulk of the force going just one mile inland. After 24hr all the units involved were back with the Seventh Fleet, having left

US Army UH-60A Black Hawks carrying members of the 82nd Airborne Brigade worked alongside Egyptian helicopters and ground forces.

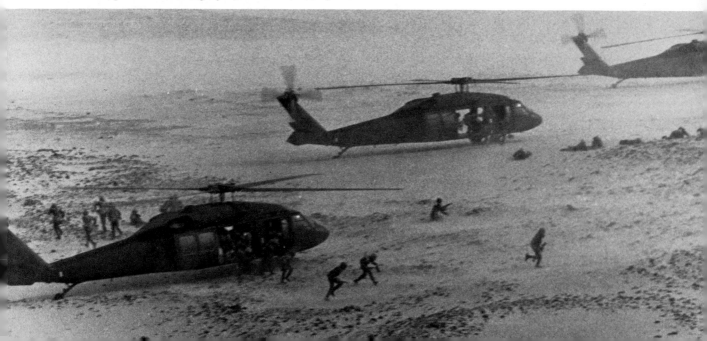

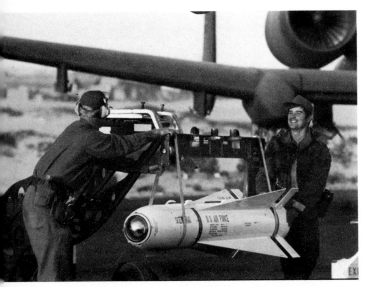

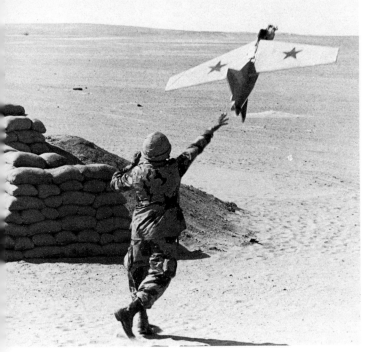

Top **Arming an A-10A with a Maverick missile.**

Above **Launching a small target drone during Bright Star 82.**

their beach-head just south of Salalah. For the Americans it was something of an anti-climax, though they were still able to demonstrate their capabilities only a few miles from the border with South Yemen.

By December 16 the last American units had left Egypt and Bright Star 82 had come to an end. Both sides had learned a lot. Flying helicopters low through sand clouds had proved damaging, the rotor blade tips soon becoming dangerously worn, especially on the smaller helicopters (the larger UH-60A Black Hawks were not so prone to this problem). Front-line servicing crews partly overcame the problem by applying tape to the worn areas, though in continuous combat this would be of doubtful efficacy. For the troops on the ground it was the discovery that their carefully designed camouflaged combat suits not only stood out against the terrain but shrank after use to cause much personal discomfort, together with the unsatisfactory design of their boots. Water proved a pressing problem, each US soldier carrying only two pints of water with him in his personal kit. Recent research has revealed that to keep active and combat-ready each man requires eight pints a day; how this requirement is to be met has yet to be worked out. The production of the water itself is no problem to the US Army, for in Somalia they successfully demonstrated a 600gal/hr salt-water purification unit.

The exercise post-mortem will go on for a long time yet, and it is to be hoped that the lessons learned will be acted upon. Apart from the fact that the RDF is now an important part of US strategy, there is the cost of Bright Star 82 itself to justify. The exercise cost a cool $60 million, the build-up phase alone requiring 450 transport flights, most of them by C-5As and C-141s. One thing is obvious, however: to make such long-range operation feasible the long tail behind the combat troops must be reduced to a more reasonable level. Although the notion of taking the American way of life into battle must be under strict review, this attitude is so entrenched that the admirable military attributes of improvisation and flexibility are in great danger of extinction. If the RDF has to be used for real, time will not be on its side. As one Israeli officer has remarked, Bright Star 82 took six months just to plan, far longer than any Middle East war has ever lasted.

Heletele is Watching You

PHILIP JARRETT

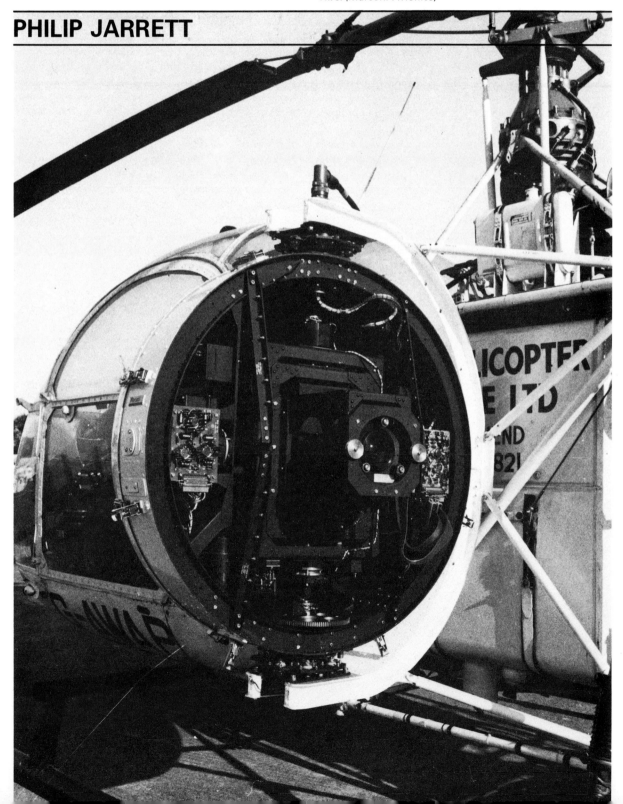

Heletele installation on an Alouette II operated by Helicopter Hire. *(Marconi Avionics)*

Have you ever appeared on television? Think carefully before you answer, because you may not have been aware of it at the time. You may have been stuck in a traffic jam, or at a large open-air public event. Were you aware of a helicopter overhead? If so, it is quite likely that it was monitoring the area with Marconi Avionics' Heletele filming and surveillance system, which is winning increasing orders from private organisations, armies, and police and security forces in the United Kingdom, the Middle East and the European continent.

Used for crowd control, film-making, traffic control and border surveillance, Heletele comprises a gimbal-mounted colour television camera, or other sensor, carried in a special spherical mounting fixed on the outside of a helicopter and controlled from within the aircraft. A data link to fixed or mobile ground stations allows events or scenes to be viewed as they happen, or recorded for analysis or editing later. Other applications include beach and coastal patrol, and surveying.

Available in day and night versions, Heletele is designed for use on small and medium helicopters. Production began at Marconi Avionics' Electro-Optical Surveillance Division, Basildon, England, seven years ago. Installations have now been developed for nine different types of European and US helicopters: the Aérospatiale Puma and Alouette II (illustrated), Agusta-Bell 212, Bell Helicopter Textron 222, Messerschmitt-Bolkow-Blöhm BO105, and the Westland Scout, Wessex 2, Whirlwind and Lynx. A typical commercial customer is the British company Helicopter Hire of Southend, Essex. Its Alouette II is hired by a wide range of organisations, including television companies.

Originally produced for the United Kingdom's Ministry of Defence, Heletele has been developed continuously to increase its versatility and usefulness. For example, not only can ground stations be reached at long range (40-60km; 25-37 miles) or short (up to 10km; 6.2 miles), but improved aerial systems and a range of viewing sensors including daylight and low-light-level television and thermal imaging are also available.

Heletele's most outstanding attribute is its exceptionally stable picture transmission, the main reason for its adoption for numerous applications. Despite the inevitable motion and vibration associated with helicopter operations, an object such as a vehicle 2km (1.25 miles) from the camera can be identified in its transmitted picture. This degree of stability permits the use of a remotely controlled zoom lens, operating over a field of view variable from 1° to 20°, which provides clear pictures at high magnification.

Space: The Last Battleground

REGINALD TURNILL

The excitement generated by the successful launch of America's Space Shuttle on its 300-mission programme over the next decade, and by the Soviet Union's new Salyut 7, aimed at providing the basis for a permanent 6/12-man space station, has stimulated much speculation about the imminence of a space war. Visions of a new breed of test pilots of the quality of Chuck Yeager and Neil Armstrong, skilfully manoeuvring their space vehicles in orbit, dodging enemy missiles and shooting down their antagonists with squirts of dazzling green laser beams, make good Biggles-type reading, and may even be fulfilled one day. But not this century.

The ability to generate powerful laser beams, point them accurately at targets hundreds or even thousands of kilometres away, and then dwell on them long enough to burn them to destruction *is* being developed by both sides, but another ten years of work is needed. In America there is continuing argument about what the US Air Force's Space Division calls the "Laser Triad," and how much money should be spent on speeding up the research.

There is no intention, I have been assured, of using the Space Shuttle as a space fighter; the next decade will be fully occupied with the more urgent task of catching

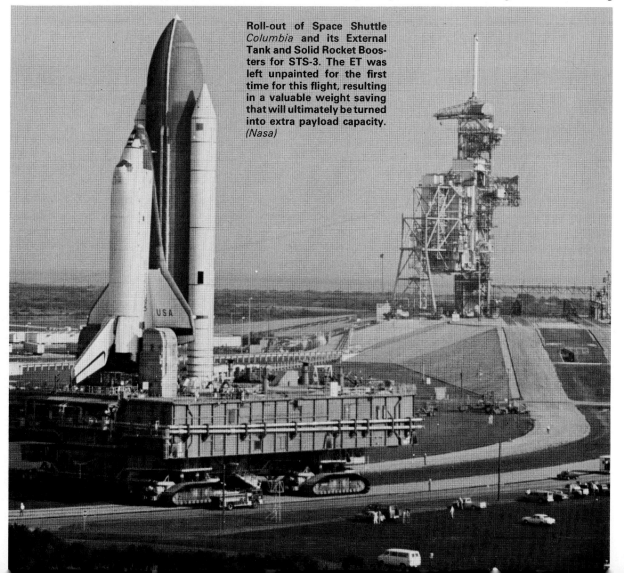

Roll-out of Space Shuttle *Columbia* and its External Tank and Solid Rocket Boosters for STS-3. The ET was left unpainted for the first time for this flight, resulting in a valuable weight saving that will ultimately be turned into extra payload capacity. (Nasa)

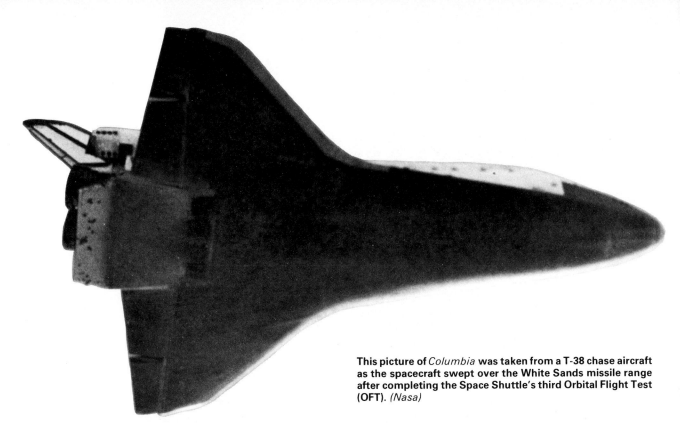

This picture of *Columbia* was taken from a T-38 chase aircraft as the spacecraft swept over the White Sands missile range after completing the Space Shuttle's third Orbital Flight Test (OFT). *(Nasa)*

up with the much delayed routine work in space. This includes using the Shuttle to deliver and service military satellites, and to conduct orbital tests of sensors and other advanced equipment for new programmes. The latter do of course include laser and particle-beam weapons, ultimately expected to be both ground and space-based.

Out of the 72 Shuttle missions planned up to 1987, 25 will include what are called DoD (Department of Defense) payloads. The first such mission involved the testing of advanced sensors on STS-4, the final Shuttle test flight, in the summer of 1982. For the first time, space correspondents covering a manned flight were not allowed to see or hear much of what was going on. But it is known that the subjects of the tests were second-generation infra-red sensors for use from about 1988 on a new series of satellites able to track selected targets anywhere in the world.

The Pentagon's own astronauts
Perhaps the most unexpected development in the past year was the news that the DoD has been quietly selecting its own exclusive group of astronauts. There has been no announcement, and I had to telephone a USAF public affairs officer in Los Angeles to get the rumour confirmed. It cannot have been good news for the 78 Nasa astronauts who have been waiting and training for flights for between four and 16 years, but it seems that the military want their own specialist astronauts available to handle delicate new equipment on the ground and in space. At present the new military astronauts are being called payload specialists, the title given to Nasa's third and lowest grade of astronaut, which calls

for the minimum of training. But the very nature of their duties would suggest that if anyone is going to take over the glamorous and dangerous role of the Yeager-type test pilots of the 1950s, it will be these military astronauts. With Nasa providing the commander and pilot on all military Shuttle missions, it seems inevitable that the duties of the military astronauts will involve much spacewalking while tending the classified equipment carried in the payload bay, and supervision of the first orbital tests of laser and particle-beam weapons.

Happily, the popular assumption that these will be tests of offensive weapons are all wrong. In fact when — and if — development of the "Laser Triad" has been completed, it will reverse the West's defence strategy.

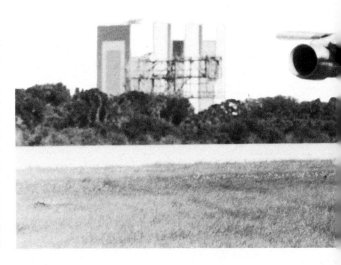

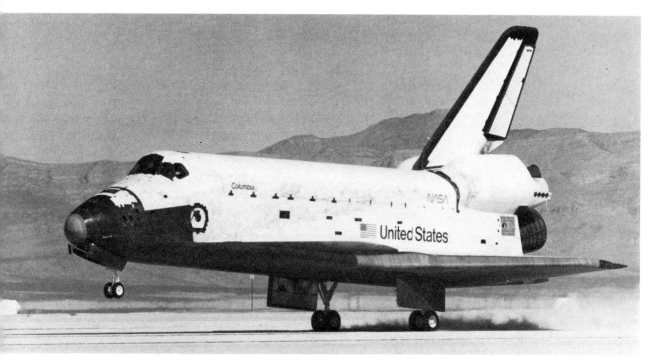

Columbia **touches down at Northrup Strip, White Sands, New Mexico, at the end of STS-3.** *(Nasa)*

The cycle completed: *Columbia* **returns after STS-3 to the Kennedy Space Centre, Cape Canaveral, atop Nasa's Boeing 747 ferry aircraft.** *(Nasa)*

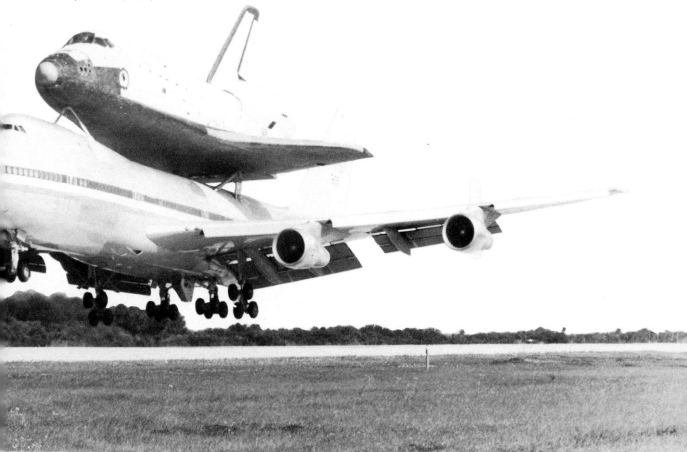

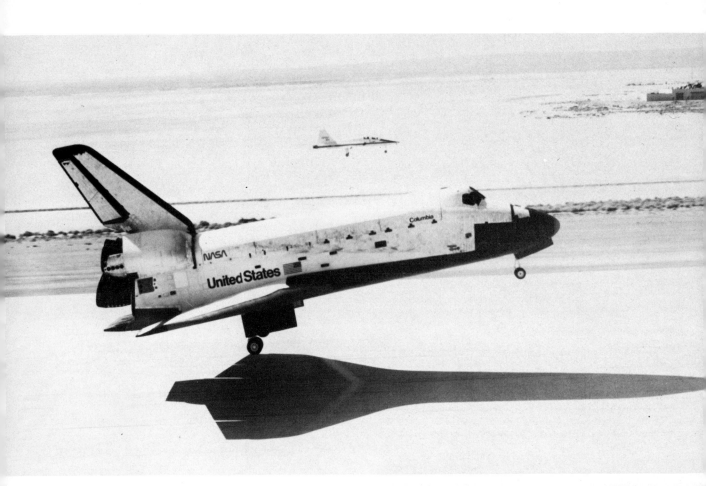

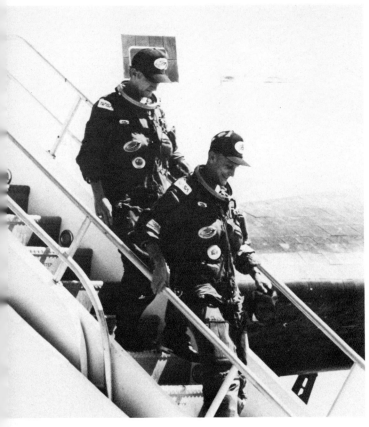

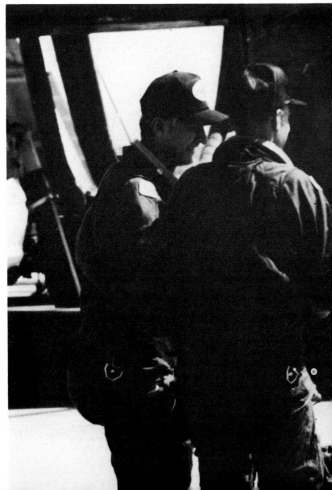

For 40 years that has been based on the concept of deterrence: having the ability to reply to any initial attack with a similar shower of nuclear-tipped missiles, thus deterring the attacker from starting a conflict because he knows that he too will be destroyed. The proposed Laser Battle Stations, as they are somewhat misleadingly called, offer at last a genuine defence against the initial attack. The present concept (which tends to change as the technology advances) is to have 24 Laser Battle Stations orbiting in three polar rings of eight at an altitude of 1,200km (745 miles). Their sensors would be capable of detecting and tracking enemy

---

Left **Throwing a Concordesque shadow,** Columbia **completes its approach to the concrete runway at Edwards AFB, California, at the end of STS-4, the final Space Shuttle test flight. This was the first time that the Orbiter had touched down on a conventional runway, presaging the planned operational round trips from Cape Canaveral and Vandenberg AFB. An uncharacteristic reluctance to tell all about the flight also reminded observers that it carried the Shuttle's first, highly secret, military payload.** (Nasa)

Below left **STS-4 astronauts Thomas Mattingly (right), a veteran of the Apollo 16 Moon flight, and Henry Hartsfield disembark from** Columbia. **Note the airline-style steps: the days when America's returned astronauts had to wait helplessly for rescuing frogmen are long gone.** (Nasa)

Below **Mattingly and Hartsfield are greeted on their return by President Reagan and his wife Nancy. Disappointment awaited those Nasa officials who had hoped that the President would use this July 4 occasion to announce funding for a fifth Orbiter and a US space station programme.** (Nasa)

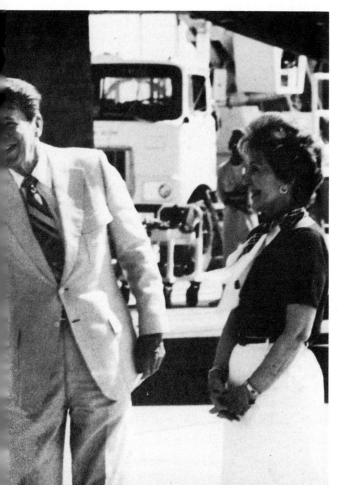

missiles the moment they were fired, and of destroying them with chemical lasers in the first four minutes of flight so that their nuclear debris fell back upon the territory of the attacker. But an indication of how far off this splendid defence capability may be is the fact that the lasers would have to deal in those four minutes with 1,000 missiles at distances of 5,000km (3,100 miles).

Effective against missiles and aircraft

Once the system had been set up it would be able to deal equally effectively with land-based and submarine-launched missiles, and with bomber, surveillance and early-warning aircraft as well. For all this, formation of a US Space Force, effectively a fourth arm of America's military services, seems inevitable in the next few years.

But with 47 Nasa Space Shuttle flights, in addition to the 25 military missions, now due by 1987, this review of the space year would be incomplete without a look at the civil effort. STS-5, the Shuttle's first operational flight, set for November 1982, is tasked with delivering two spacecraft into low earth orbit so that they can be fired from there into synchronous orbits. One of them, SBS-C, is for America's Satellite Business Systems, a commercial communications system with the incredible ability to transmit a column of business data the size of Tolstoy's War and Peace anywhere in the world in just one second. The other, Telesat-E, will provide Canada with TV and voice communications.

The first US woman astronaut has been chosen, out of turn as we predicted last year, to fly on STS-7, due for launch on April 20, 1983. Dr Sally Ride, who is a physicist, earned her place by becoming expert in the use of the robot arm — officially called the Remote Manipulator System — and by proving her competence during both STS-2 and STS-3 during spells as capcom (a rather out of date term meaning "capsule communicator"), passing instructions and advice to the crews in orbit.

Busy mission for first US spacewoman

On what is planned as a six-day flight in Challenger, the second Space Shuttle Orbiter, Sally will have a much busier time than world's first spacewoman Valentina Tereshkova in her first-generation capsule. Not only will STS-7 be orbiting two more satellites, for Canada and Indonesia, but it is hoped to carry out a rehearsal for the first attempt at repairing a damaged satellite in orbit. The Solar Maximum Mission spacecraft, launched into a 500km (310-mile) orbit in February 1980 to study solar flares and help us to understand how the Sun works, blew its fuses ten months later and has been of little use since. The plan now is to take Columbia alongside in December 1983, grab SMM with the robot arm, pull it into the cargo bay, repair it, and then replace it in orbit so that it can start its work again.

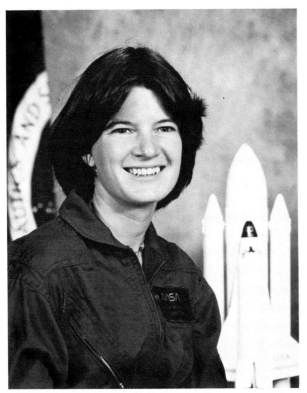

Sally Ride, America's first woman astronaut. She is due to fly on STS-7, currently scheduled for April 1983, and is expected to be followed at intervals by the other seven women at present undergoing astronaut training. *(Nasa)*

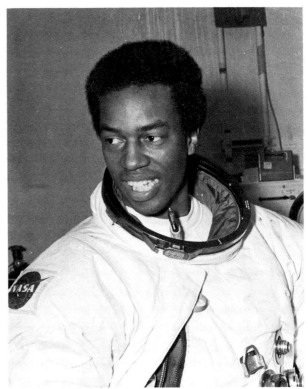

Guion Bluford, Vietnam veteran and now set to become America's first black astronaut. He is due to fly on STS-8 in July 1983. *(Nasa)*

We have been given no details yet as to how these complicated manoeuvres can be rehearsed, but clearly a lot of delicate manipulation with the robot arm will be called for, as well as spacewalking. It is an open secret at Nasa (the male astronauts discourage its discussion!) that the women have shown a more delicate touch in working the robot arm, so this may well prove to be Sally's big chance. As a mission specialist she could also become the first woman to do an EVA, though that seems unlikely on this flight. Robert Crippen, who flew on STS-1 as No 2 to John Young, will be commander on STS-7, while none of the other three crew members has flown before. The pilot will be Fred Hauk, a US Navy commander, and the other mission specialist will be Dr John Fabian, a lieutenant-colonel in the US Air Force specialising in aeronautical engineering. All three were selected as astronauts in Group 8 only four years ago, so there must be some long faces among the veterans still awaiting their first flight.

The first black astronaut
There must have been similar dismay about STS-8, a three-day mission due in July 1983, which will give Richard Truly, pilot on STS-2, his first command. His three-man crew are also comparative youngsters from Group 8, and will include Guion Bluford, who will have the distinction of becoming the first black astronaut.

Yet another surprise was the announcement that John Young, the only man to have made five spaceflights, intends to clock up his sixth and celebrate his 53rd birthday in orbit as STS-9 commander on the all-important first Spacelab mission in September. At the end of STS-1, Suzy, his much relieved wife, said repeatedly that if she had anything to do with it, he would never go into space again. Five times on top of those rockets was quite enough risk for anyone, especially their wives, she insisted. But the seven-day Spacelab flight, with the first six-astronaut crew, is of great international importance: Spacelab was developed by ten member countries of the European Space Agency, and will be carrying as a payload specialist the first European astronaut to fly in a Western vehicle, plus US and European experiments.

The drive to save weight
Government budget cuts have made international collaboration increasingly important to Nasa. Its only hope of going ahead with construction of a permanent space station in an effort to catch up with the Soviet Union in this field is to persuade the European Space Agency, Canada and, perhaps, Japan to join in and share the cost. Equally important is an increase in the efficiency of the Space Shuttle system, which at present is costing much more than was originally hoped. It still takes a 2,000-ton cluster of rockets to place less than 30

tons of satellite and equipment in orbit. A long-term programme to reduce the total lift-off weight, and so increase the payload by roughly the same amount, is therefore under way. The change in colour of the External Tank from STS-2's gleaming white to the light brown STS-3 was evidence of the first small step in this direction: a 27kg (60lb) weight reduction was achieved by leaving off the white paint. Many other changes to reduce the weight of both the ET and the Solid Rocket Boosters are in hand. Martin Marietta, which makes the ET, has proposed that on STS-7 *Challenger*, instead of jettisoning the tank just before going into orbit, should carry it on into orbit. An astronaut — it could be Sally Ride — would use the Manned Mobility Unit to make a fly-around inspection of the ET and find out how much insulation it really needs during launch. There could be many bonuses from such an operation. First and foremost, Martin Marietta thinks that the weight of the ET could be reduced by many tons, permanently improving the performance of the Shuttle, reducing launch costs and

making it more competitive with the rival launcher, ESA's Ariane. It would be the first time an astronaut had carried out an EVA without a tether, and would increase confidence that repairs, like that planned for the Solar Maximum spacecraft, could be carried out in orbit. Finally, it would demonstrate the feasibility of taking the huge External Tanks into orbit and leaving them there for future use as building blocks for space stations.

All this would pave the way for a colourful conclusion to 1983, rivalling in drama the famous round-the-Moon flight of Christmas 1968. The four-astronaut crew of STS-11 is due to lift off on December 23, 1983, and spend the next five days carrying out the first spacecraft retrieval and repair operation. Success would have profound significance for man's future in space, speeding up many different sorts of orbital activities. One hopes that those activities will mainly be peaceful ones, like the production of much improved vaccines for medical use, but they could also have military applications.

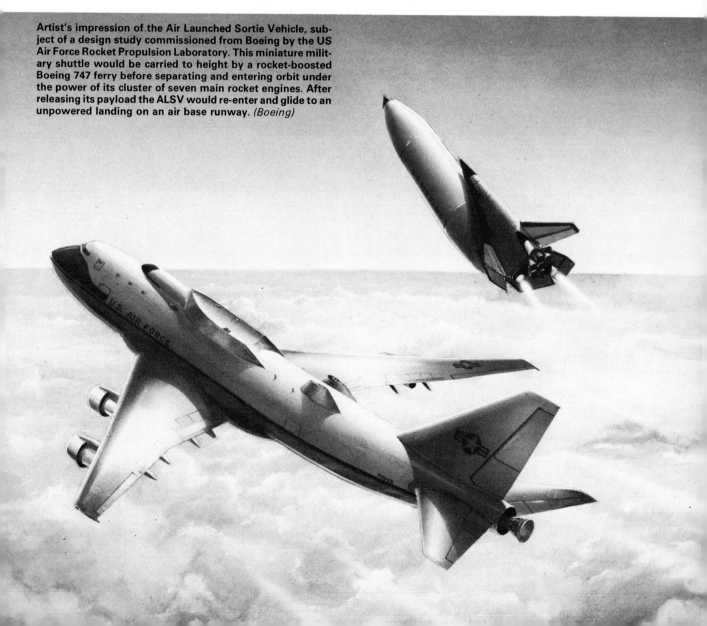

Artist's impression of the Air Launched Sortie Vehicle, subject of a design study commissioned from Boeing by the US Air Force Rocket Propulsion Laboratory. This miniature military shuttle would be carried to height by a rocket-boosted Boeing 747 ferry before separating and entering orbit under the power of its cluster of seven main rocket engines. After releasing its payload the ALSV would re-enter and glide to an unpowered landing on an air base runway. *(Boeing)*

SHUTTLE FLIGHT LOG

Mission	Launch date	Crew	Orbits	Duration (days, hr, min)	Comments
STS-1	April 12, 1981	John Young Robert Crippen	36	02.06.21	Near-perfect first flight
STS-2	November 12, 1981	Joe Engle Richard Truly	36	02.06.13	Five-day mission halved by fuel-cell fault
STS-3	March 22, 1982	Jack Lousma Charles Fullerton	129	08.00.05	Extra day because of storm at Northrup
STS-4	June 27, 1982	Thomas Mattingly Henry Hartsfield	119	07.11.00	Last OFT verifying hardware and software systems
STS-5	November 1982	Vance Brand Robert Overmyer Joseph Allen William Lenoir			Five-day first operational mission. First flight for mission specialists
STS-6	January 1983	Paul Weitz Karol Bobko Donald Peterson Story Musgrave			First flight of *Challenger*. Two days, to deploy TDRS-1
STS-7	April 1983	Robert Crippen Frederick Hauk Sally Ride John Fabian			First US woman astronaut. Possible SMM repair rehearsal with ET in orbit
STS-8	July 1983	Richard Truly Daniel Brandenstein Guion Bluford Dale Gardner			Two days, to deploy TDRS-2 and India's Insat 1B
STS-9	September 1983	John Young Brewster Shaw Owen Garriott Robert Parker + two payload specialists			Spacelab 1
STS-10	November 1983				Classified DoD mission
STS-11	December 1983				SMM repair mission

Gee Bee Reborn

BILL TURNER

Whenever aviation enthusiasts gather to talk about aeroplanes, catastrophes or engineering advances, there is always one name that is spoken in almost reverent tones: Gee Bee. Such is the mystique surrounding the handful of racing aircraft produced in Springfield, Massachusetts, by the Granville Brothers Aircraft Company. In their teens and twenties these young men (only two of the five with a completed high school education), aided and abetted by engineers Bob Hall and Pete Miller, changed the course of aviation history with their innovative machines.

When the first of their great thundering, roaring racers made its spectacular debut in 1931, its top speed bettered that of the fastest fighter in the world by more than 160km/hr (100mph). The Model Z — or "Number Four," as the Granville brothers always referred to it — burst upon the aviation scene like a meteor. The stubby prodigy was entered for and won five races, including the prestigious Thompson Trophy, unofficially shattered the landplane speed record and then disappeared in a ball of fire — all in just 90 days.

Replica Gee Bee Model Z *City of Springfield,* **built by Bill Turner and Ed Marquart.** *(Howard Levy)*

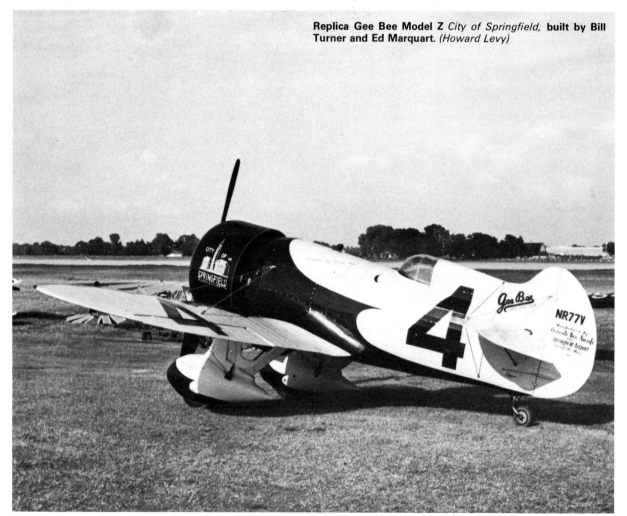

I chose the Model Z for resurrection because it is by far the most historically significant of the Granville products. Working very closely with me and the man who did most of the building, Ed Marquart, were the two surviving Granville brothers, Bob and Ed. Both supplied a wealth of information, Ed spending a great deal of time in California to ensure that an exact copy of the original would result. Their constant attention to detail can never again be applied to the recreation of any further Gee Bees for both died before the Model Z replica flew. Bob missed it by only ten days.

All but one of the five Gee Bee racers met their end during take-off or landing. My replica of Number Four is no exception. The Model Z touches down at 153km/hr (95mph) in a three-point attitude. The tiny rudder is immediately useless for guidance down the runway, and hard braking is required for control. On that fateful day in June 1979, at Half Moon Bay, California, the brakes failed completely and the Model Z darted off the runway, tripped itself in soft sand and flipped over onto its back. My time on the Gee Bee is greater than the combined total of all the pilots who flew the tricky racers in the 1930s, and I lived to add to it, surviving the crash with cuts, bruises and a bad shaking up. Happily, the Gee Bee is back to flying status and is currently on loan to the city museum at Springfield, Massachusetts, birthplace of the original aeroplanes.

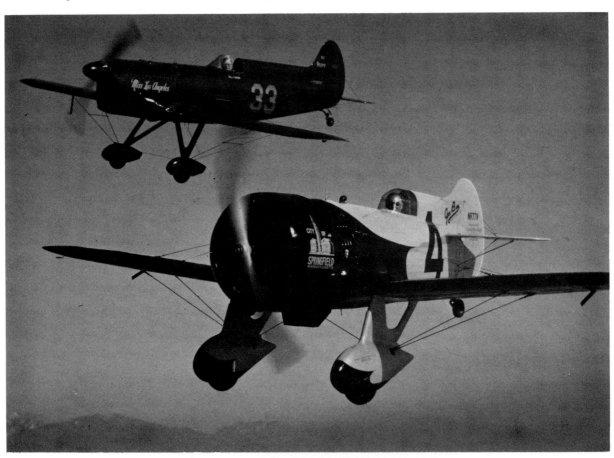

Bill Turner's Gee Bee flying alongside his Brown Racer Miss Los Angeles **over Riverside, California.**

Little Nellie and the Wallis Sisters

Wg Cdr K. H. WALLIS

Mention the Wallis autogyros and most people call to mind James Bond's *Little Nellie*, the diminutive but deadly reconnaissance aircraft featured in the film *You Only Live Twice*. However, *Little Nellie* was not the first Wallis autogyro to break into films. The 1961 prototype, G-ARRT, was heard but not seen in *Those Magnificent Men in their Flying Machines* when she was made to misfire while flying over recording equipment. The resulting sound effects were used throughout the film.

In 1966 G-ARRT won a star role in an Italian film to be shot in Brazil and Italy. An interview by Tony Scase on the planned filming was broadcast on the BBC's *Today* programme, which in turn was heard by the art director of the Bond film, then in the making. A demonstration of an autogyro at Pinewood Studios was

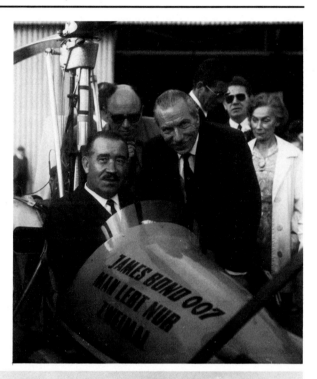

Wing Commander K. H. Wallis (standing) shows the diminutive *Little Nellie* to General Adolf Galland, the German fighter ace of the Second World War. *(Horst Janke)*

G-ARRT in 1969, after gaining the 3km speed record for autogyros, beside the Harrier that had just set a new London-New York centre-to-centre record. *(Crown Copyright)*

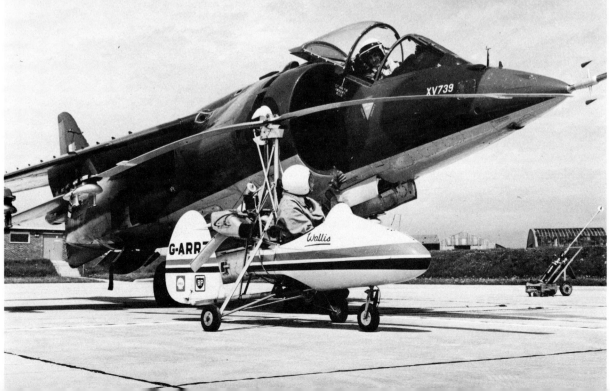

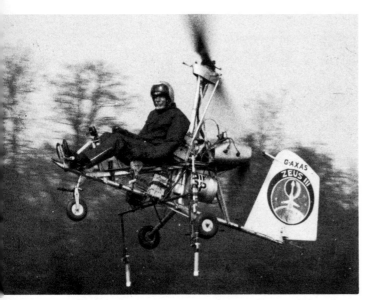

WA-116-T/Mc G-AXAS pictured during filming of *The Martian Chronicles.*

urgently requested, and along went the ex-military Beagle-Wallis WA-116 XR943, then demobbed as G-ARZB. The demonstration resulted in a part in the film. I then went to Brazil, as originally planned, to fly G-ARRT over the dramatic mountains near Rio de Janeiro, before going on to the volcanic area of Southern Japan, where *Little Nellie* was to win her aerial battles. She and her older sister had become stars.

The two-seater G-AXAS has also had a film part, playing in the production of Ray Bradbury's *The Martian Chronicles*, shot on Malta and the Canary Islands. On such film work the autogyros are also used to carry film cameras, up to 35mm Panavision size, to record the pilot's point of view. Take-offs and landings often have to be made at very small sites, while the filming may require flying over and in volcano craters at 1,830m (6,000ft). Film-making is hard and exacting work, and fun only when it is completed.

Since becoming a star *Little Nellie* has also become an exhibitionist, demonstrating her attributes in public at over 500 displays in fifteen countries. Her sister G-AXAS has lately taken to the reputedly dangerous practice of hitching lifts on moving lorries. Happily, both sisters can look after themselves, and G-AXAS is as adept at jumping off the lorry as she is at dropping in. G-AXAS has also shown her ability to land on a moving ship, alighting on the pleasure boat *Solent Scene*.

The experiments with moving vehicles were actually some of the more serious test roles for this minimal two-seater. From the outset the Wallis autogyros were designed with military, police and similar roles in view. As early as 1962-3, three Beagle-Wallis autogyros were tested by the British Army. They proved capable of performing many tasks normally carried out at much greater cost by aeroplanes or helicopters, and in many roles they even proved superior. The special attributes of the autogyro are: extremely small size and easy road transportability; the ability to fly trimmed hands-off for long periods, even in turbulence, leaving the pilot to concentrate on a primary task; safe operation at low altitudes and speeds, as they always fly in the emergency mode of a helicopter, auto-rotation; low vibration level; unequalled field of view; and absence of rotor downwash, which at low speeds and altitudes would reduce the effectiveness of sensors and destroy or disperse evidence.

The lack of a really suitable engine has been the chief bar to production for military and serious commercial use. However, while the long search for the right engine continues, the various Wallis autogyros have been operated usefully for 21 years. Some of the useful

G-AXAS lands on a moving lorry.

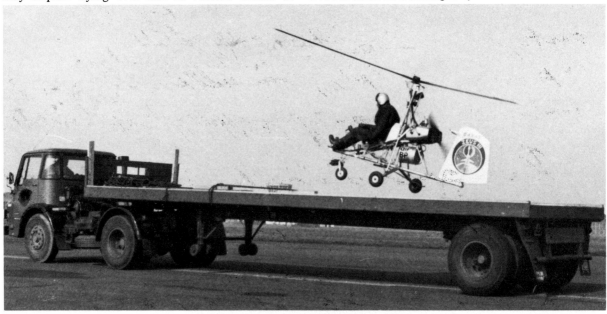

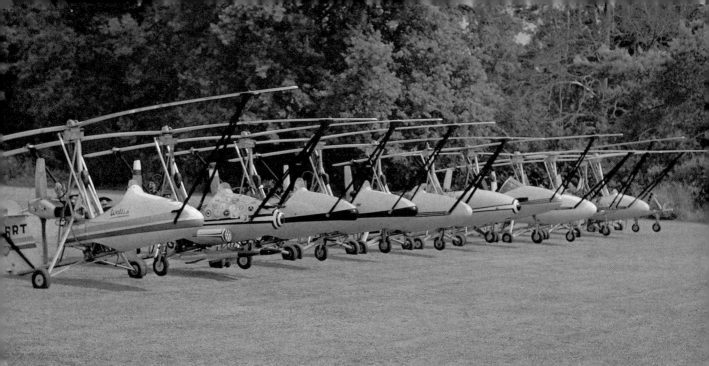

1980 line-up of the Wallis sisters, less the WA-120.

work lies in the formal testing of the aircraft and in proof-of-performance world record flights, both of which contribute greatly to the understanding of rotary-winged flight. Many roles have been purely operational, however, and some of this work is described below. (The suffix behind each aircraft type number denotes the engine fitted; e.g. Mc denotes McCulloch, F denotes Franklin).

WA-116/Mc (G-ARRT)
As early as 1961 this prototype was in use as a photographic platform, sometimes for pure photography and

WA-116/F G-ASDY in original form in 1963.

on other occasions for aircraft test recordings. Helmet-mounted and fixed 16mm cine cameras were used, backing up strain-gauging and performance trials for certification. More advanced photography followed, with large-format F-24 aerial reconnaissance cameras being used for coastal ecology research and the survey of archaeological sites. Returning briefly to performance testing in 1968-9, G-ARRT broke the auto-gyro world records for altitude and speed.

WA-116/Fs (G-ASDY, G-ATHL, G-ATHM and XR944)
G-ASDY, the fourth military WA-116/Mc, was built in 1962. For years she was something of a "hack," used to introduce pilots to autogyros and for experiments. Rig-

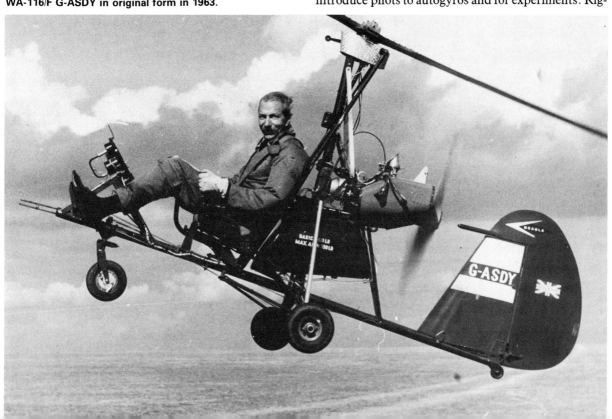

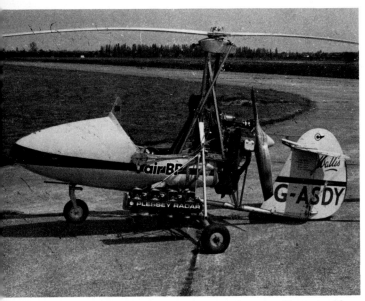

G-ASDY fitted with a multi-band photographic pack of four cameras for the detection of hidden objects.

G-ASDY in 1978, with a Vinten Type 360 oblique camera. (Brian M. Lane)

ged with high-speed cameras rotating with the rotor blades, she has been put through her paces, the cameras observing rotor dynamics and, by the wool-tuft method, aerodynamics.

In 1965 her McCulloch was replaced by a Wallis-modified Hillman Imp car engine. The object was to find an off-the-shelf engine for aero-club use. A WA-116/Mc was being used at that time by the Norfolk and Norwich Aero Club. Many pilots were flying the aircraft, but the noise of the McCulloch became as unpopular with the locals as its occasional silence did with the pilots. Performance of the "Aero-Imp" was good, but the noise of the ungeared propeller was unacceptable. Reduction gearing would have increased weight and added complication. G-ASDY therefore languished in water-cooled solitude until, in 1971, the Imp engine was replaced by a 44.7kW (60hp) Franklin two-cylinder aero engine. It was immediately apparent that this airframe/engine combination was right. Cruise performance was excellent, and the low exhaust note and noise intensity were acceptable to public and pilot.

G-ASDY started a new career thereafter, and has been much in demand for multi-band photographic and other remote-sensing tasks. In collaboration with the Plessey Radar Research Centre the aircraft has been

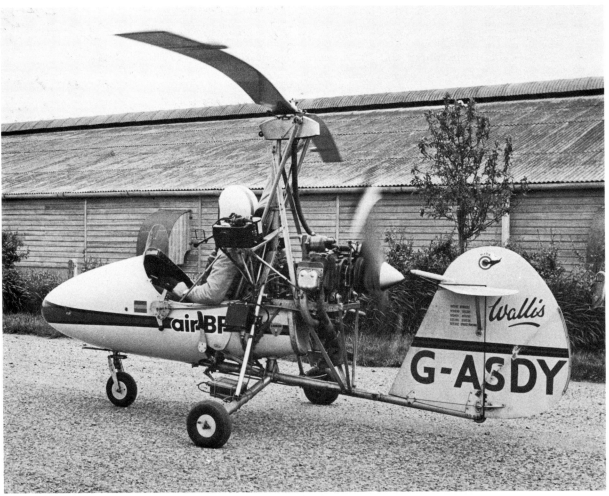

used for Home Office trials and police operations, mainly in connection with the detection of illicit graves. Electronics experiments have entailed the carriage of a large aerial array which has to be extended below the lowest part of the aircraft in flight. The array was made in two halves and hinged so that it could be moved to the sides of the aircraft and upwards for take-offs and landings.

In 1981 G-ASDY completed a colour stereo-photographic survey of the Broadlands area of Norfolk and Suffolk in three two-hour flights. The work was for the Institute of Terrestrial Ecology and was undertaken with a vertical Vinten Type 360 reconnaissance camera with 6in lens and automatic exposure control.

This first Franklin-engined WA-116 showed that further improvements could still be made. A quiet, reliable and economical engine had long been awaited before making serious attacks on the autogyro world records for distance, speed over distance, and duration. WA-116/Mc G-ATHM was chosen for this role. Built in 1965 and operated on a tea plantation in Ceylon as 4R-ACK, she returned to the family in 1970.

Conversion work started on January 1, 1974. In July she flew non-stop more than five times the previous 100km closed-circuit record distance and set the first 500km closed-circuit speed records for autogyros. That flight gave some indication of her potential, leading to a non-stop flight from Lydd, Kent, to Wick, Caithness, via Inverness and various air traffic diversions. The distance flown, in a crosswind, was some 965km (600 miles), at an average speed of 150km/hr (93mph). On landing there was fuel for a further hour of flight.

This aircraft is useful for long-range photographic work because of its ability to journey some distance especially when road transportation of aircraft and equipment to the site is not convenient. An example of this was the filming for a TV documentary of the 7.10 a.m. train from Yarmouth to London. It was possible to stay in bed a little longer but still be over Yarmouth to record the train pulling out of the station, and then be at various places en route. On another occasion a TV documentary necessitated filming "duck's eye" views of landings and take-offs from a tree-encircled duck decoy in Suffolk.

Other WA-116/Mc airframes have now been converted to the thoroughly practical F version. A recent example is again wearing the military uniform of XR944, one of the Army versions, and she was seen at the Army Air Corps Centre during celebrations of the 25th anniversary of the Corps.

Unfortunately, Franklin has ceased manufacture. However, there is now a new British engine of much the same size and configuration. Incorporating the latest combustion chamber techniques in which its manufacturer specialises, the Weslake should be a more powerful and economical unit for the planned production version of the WA-116 airframe.

The military XR944 in latest WA-116/F form.

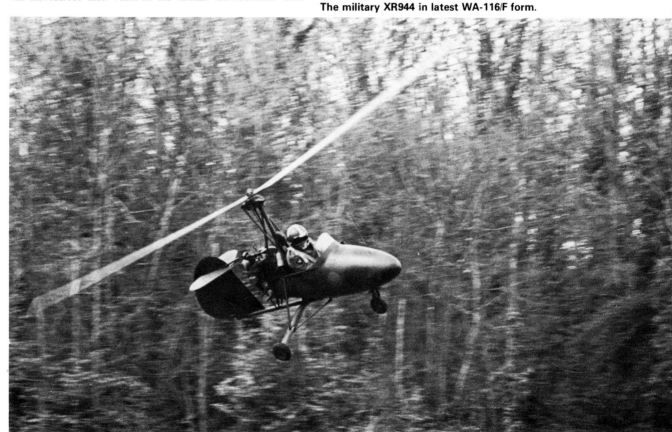

WA-117/R-R Series 2 (G-AVJV)

The long search for the right engine naturally included trials with the 74.5kW (100hp) Rolls-Royce/Continental O-200. The first WA-117 was G-ATCV. The design envisaged an advanced, fully enclosed and semi-reclining cockpit. To allow space for a suitably large-diameter two-blade propeller the keel was cranked and the rudder was supported at the keel and from an extension below the rotor head. Flight tests before fitting the cockpit nacelle suggested that this design was a retrograde step. The aircraft was dismantled and the parts used to build the WA-117 Series 2, an aircraft much more on the lines of a WA-116 and registered G-AVJV. The result was what might be described as a very "quiet and respectable sister", a really hard-working girl.

The quietness of G-AVJV resulted from the use of a small-diameter four-blade propeller with low tip speed, and engine exhaust silencing. Sound recording equipment was used for trials in Norfolk, but G-AVJV was so nearly silent that she caused no increase in the ambient noise level at a vertical range of 1,070 m (3,500ft) and a slant range of 915m (3,000ft). This meant that the autogyro was quiet enough to be used to patrol Loch Ness in the summer of 1970, assisting the Loch Ness Investigation Bureau in the search for the monster. "Nessie" did not deign to appear for aerial photography, but it was a useful exercise of a type in which the aircraft excels.

The same year G-AVJV was equipped with the

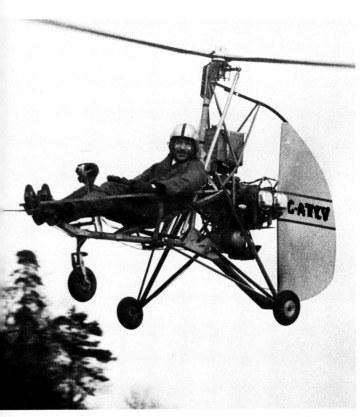

WA-117/R-R in Series 1 form in 1965, during early trials without the cockpit nacelle.

WA-117/R-R Series 2 in 1970, with Hawker Siddeley Dynamics infra-red Linescan.

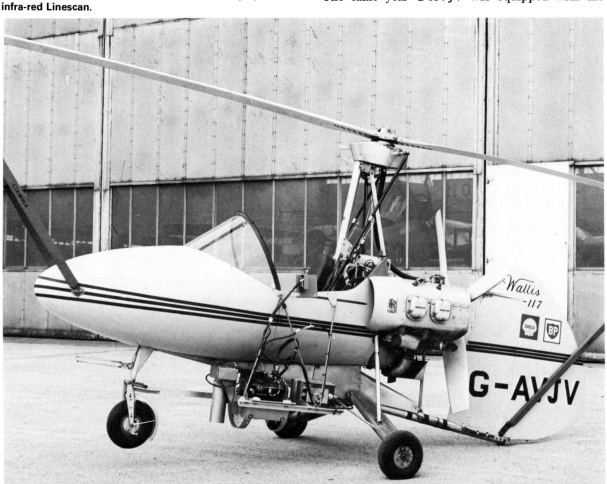

Hawker Siddeley Dynamics infra-red Linescan and operated at night over the Bovingdon tank training area. Take-offs and landings were made at a playing field by the lights of a car, a technique perfected with the WA-116 prototype (G-ARRT) some years before. Other work with G-AVJV has entailed the use of large-format cameras, including a special Wallis adaptation to provide continuous-strip photography of the ground overflown.

Video work started in 1970 and continues to date. Before the aircraft could be used for such work acceptable vibration levels had to be proved. This was done at night, using an open-shutter F-24 camera and a "chopped" light source on the ground to determine the vibration characteristics. Much other testing has been done, recording pitch attitude over a wide speed range, and checking control response and stability. Control input transducers and three-axis rate gyros were fitted, the resulting data being stored on an Admiralty recorder.

'JV has been used almost continuously for multi-spectral and multi-band photography. This started with coastal ecology research at Dungeness. Later a refined system was used in connection with Plessey Radar Research and in police searches for buried corpses. For some of these tasks very accurate height-keeping was essential, and a Plessey radar altimeter became part of the equipment. Carrying a British Aerospace Dynamics Linescan Type 213, and a false-colour infra-red camera, the aircraft has been successfully used to detect leaks in water pipelines 2.4m (8ft) underground.

Photography by "narrow-cut red filtration" of a site on Hayling Island, described on the Ordnance Survey maps as a Roman villa, will necessitate a change in the map: the "villa" turned out to be a temple.

Many will have seen the dramatic pictures of central London exhibited at the 1978 SBAC Show and taken with the Vinten Type 751 panoramic camera. These were taken from WA-117 G-AVJV, as were a number of shots for television. These included the Harwich-Hook of Holland ferry leaving harbour and at sea, and the Thames barge race off Southend. For the latter task only an autogyro is acceptable, since there is no rotor downwash to affect the sails.

WA-120/R-R (G-AYVO)

First flown in 1971, before the Franklin engine was fitted to a WA-116, G-AYVO was built as a long-range autogyro. With a fully enclosed cockpit, 73lit (16 Imp gal) internal fuel tank and an economical Rolls-Royce O-240 engine of 97kW (130hp), she could have been in the record-breaking business. However, the smaller and lighter WA-116/F was considered more appropriate for the record flights, while the greater lifting capacity of the WA-120 was exploited for specialised

WA-120/R-R G-AYVO fitted with a pack of four Vinten 70mm multi-band reconnaissance cameras.

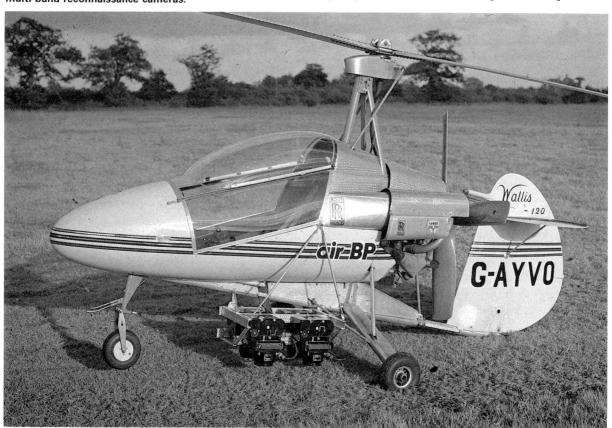

photography with a multi-band pack of four Vinten Type 360 cameras operating through narrow-band filtration. Since 1976 G-AYVO has formed part of the "Exploration" exhibition at the Science Museum. The use of the camera pack is illustrated by the pollution survey of Langstone Harbour which was conducted by the aircraft.

The two-seaters

Two open-frame two-seater Wallis autogyros are in use. One, WA-116-T/Mc G-AXAS, has already been mentioned. The experience gained with G-AXAS contributed to the design of WA-122/R-R G-BGGW. With a 97kW (130hp) Rolls-Royce engine and more room for the rear occupant, this aircraft is proving to be a very useful dual-control pilot conversion trainer. However, as with G-AXAS, the special low-speed properties of these machines when flown solo, combined with unimpaired visibility and the absence of downwash, quickly brought in other tasks. One such job was a search near Basingstoke in September 1980 for a part of the turbine disc from the McDonnell Douglas F-18 Hornet fighter prototype, which crashed after the SBAC Show. That effort was not successful, but another search did restore a valuable lost bull calf to his anxious mother!

The exotic sisters and the working girls

Only two "exotic" Wallis sisters exist at the moment. One is WA-118/M Meteorite G-AVJW. Powered by an Italian Meteor-Alfa four-cylinder supercharged radial two-stroke of 89.5kW (120hp), this rather temperamental prima donna has a very beautiful voice. At present she is waiting in the wings for a chance to demonstrate her extreme altitude capability. The other is the very small and light WA-121/Mc, intended for speed and altitude experiments when time permits. On July 20, 1982, WA-121/Mc G-BAHH attained an altitude of 5,640m (18,504ft).

Working autogyros for production

Over the last twenty years the Wallis autogyros have conclusively proved that they are capable of useful and specialised work. Serviceability has been excellent, and in the very many hundreds of working flights there has never been a take-off delayed.

Close collaboration with Weslake is about to result in an engine built for the WA-116 airframe — this is the first new British light aero-engine for decades — and a production design is now possible.

The association with aerial reconnaissance specialists W. Vinten Ltd has resulted in an agreement for licensed production of the Wallis autogyros, and the company is now CAA-approved for manufacture. The aim is to build the aircraft to meet aerial-work certification requirements and to market them for military and serious commercial roles.

WA-118/M Meteorite.

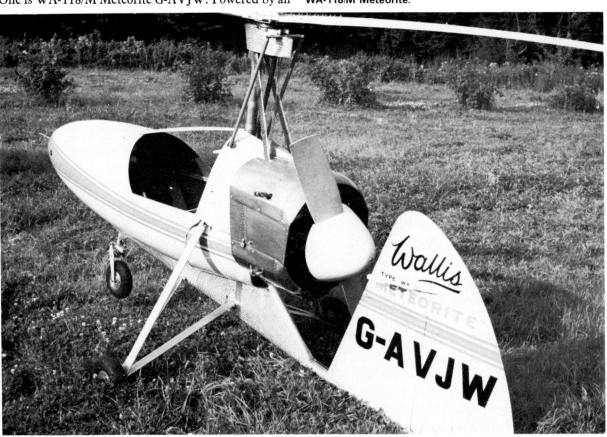

Can the Airship Come Back?

There are two ways of flying within the Earth's atmosphere: the dynamic, in heavier-than-air vehicles, and the static, using lighter-than-air craft. Both methods were probably first demonstrated by the Chinese more than two thousand years ago, though they have been used for untethered human flight only within the past two hundred years. Invention of the internal combustion engine towards the end of the last century finally produced, amost simultaneously, practical airships and aeroplanes.

US Navy non-rigid airship G-1, known as *Defender* when operated within the Goodyear fleet. Used for maritime patrol.

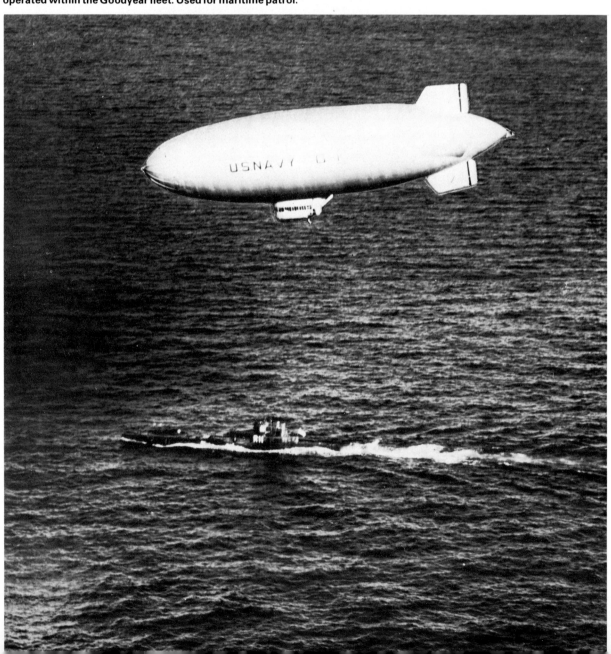

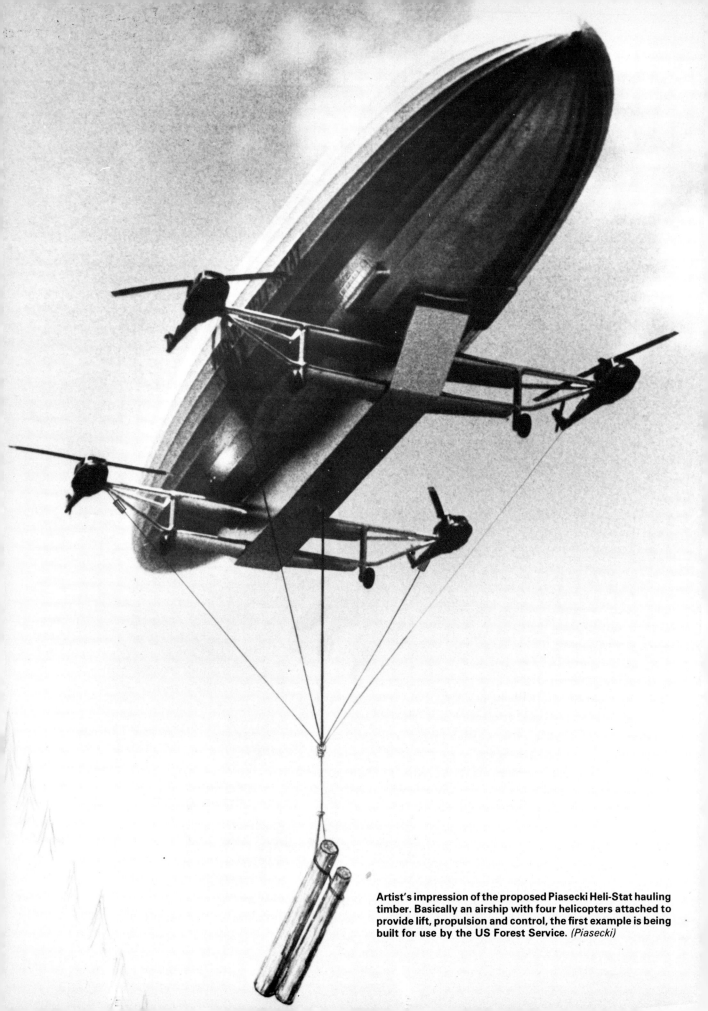

Artist's impression of the proposed Piasecki Heli-Stat hauling timber. Basically an airship with four helicopters attached to provide lift, propulsion and control, the first example is being built for use by the US Forest Service. *(Piasecki)*

Airships are of two types: rigids, with structural hulls enclosing numerous gasbags, and pressure airships (usually called blimps), in which the sustaining gas is contained directly under slight pressure in a single large envelope. The latter can be provided with a stiffening keel, in which case they are sometimes called semi-rigid. Another intermediate type is the metalclad, in which the envelope takes the form of a metal-covered structure which derives its rigidity partly from the pressure of the contained gas.

Rigids have long been regarded as the most promising type for major transport applications, and this still seems to be accepted by some of today's advocates of airships. A few of the latter also believe that the rigid should be of the metalclad type. Pressure airships, which were used extensively for inshore maritime patrol during the two world wars, are still advocated by some for this role, although their smaller lifting capacity and lower speeds are serious limitations. For the past twenty years the only types flying have been small pressure airships used for advertising and joyriding, primarily by the American Goodyear Tire and Rubber Company, which has been continuously engaged in airship manufacture and operation for nearly 65 years.

The pressure airship's initial promise early in the twentieth century soon began to fade in the face of the aeroplane's rapid development. From a status of almost equal importance during the first decade of the century, the pressure airship was seen as of only limited military value by the end of the second decade. High hopes were however still entertained for the large rigid's use as a long-haul transport, especially after the success of the German DELAG passenger-carrying airships between 1910 and 1914. These hopes were sustained through the third decade but faded during the fourth after the tragic losses of the British R101 and the German *Hindenburg*. The Second World War saw the airship having a final fling in the inshore maritime patrol role with the US Navy, but even this service had

dropped airships by 1962. Since then the world's population of airships could be counted on the fingers of one hand. Heavier-than-air aircraft, with fixed or rotary wings, have swept the board and are now unchallenged in every airborne role.

A rare species

The reasons for this are simple. Because of the low density of the atmosphere airships must be very large if they are to carry useful loads. Large size means costly development, and high manufacturing and operating costs. As that great pioneer aviation journalist C. G. Grey once said, "aeroplanes breed like rabbits, airships like elephants". There have therefore been very few of them. Small numbers mean a small spread of development costs and less benefit from the "learning curve," which brings down cost as more examples of any one design are manufactured. It also means a slower accumulation of total flying hours and operating experience. Smaller numbers also mean fewer users to spread the inevitably high cost of developing, manufacturing and operating ground facilities and all-weather operating aids, most of which would have to be specially provided for airships.

High operating costs mean that, right from the start, a lot of traffic (passengers or freight) is required on the routes operated. A smaller and less costly vehicle is much more satisfactory in maintaining an adequate frequency while traffic is gradually built up to levels that justify a larger replacement. Large size contributes also to what is perhaps the airship's greatest handicap: difficulties of handling on the ground. This is not such a problem for pressure airships, but rigids could be as large as a modern giant oil tanker. Yet at the same time it would be literally as light as a feather: an awkward

The Goodyear airship *Europa*, used by Thames Television in 1981 to take aerial photographs of the British royal wedding. *(Thames Television)*

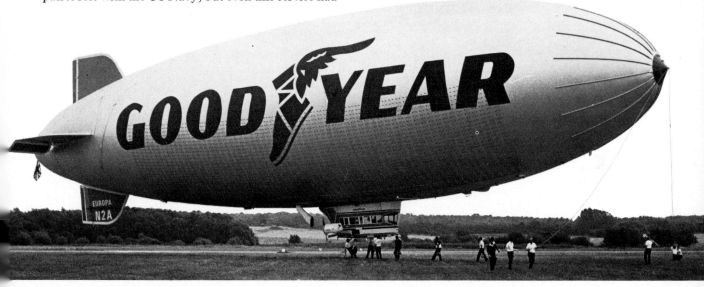

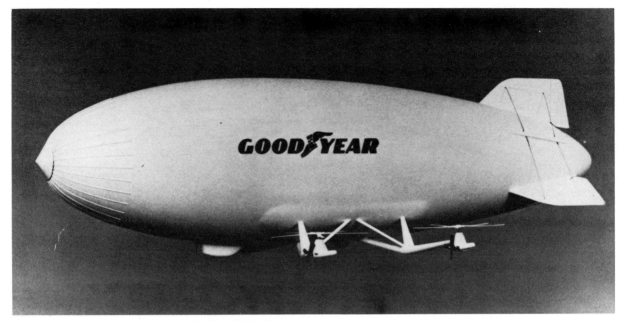

A Goodyear proposal for a heavy-lift airship with helicopter-type rotors for lift and conventional propellers for forward flight. (Goodyear)

object indeed to moor on the ground or to manhandle into a hangar in any sort of wind.

The large hull or envelope containing the lifting gas causes so much drag that speeds are low, embarrassingly so in an atmosphere which often has wind strengths equal to a high percentage of airship cruising speeds. This gives long and very variable sector times, creating difficulties when the operator is trying to maintain economic schedules with high utilisation of aircraft and crews. Aeroplane experience shows that cruising speeds of at least 150kt are required to minimise the effect of winds, and this is likely to remain outside airship capabilities in the foreseeable future.

Against this negative background, it at first appears remarkable that there have been a number of initiatives to revive airships during the twenty years since the last major airship operator, the US Navy, gave them up. These efforts have been in two areas: relatively small pressure airships, and large (often very large) rigid airships, some of metalclad type.

The airship misunderstood

Much of the publicity surrounding this work has tended to ignore the major technical differences between the two types of airship. It has suggested that relatively modest developments, starting with small blimps, provide a logical lead-in to large transport airships, usually of rigid type, requiring enormously greater industrial muscle, expensive research and development, and large financial resources. History suggests that development of such large airships would be possible only by means of a very big programme, perhaps comparable in scale and cost with current major heavier-than-air efforts. (Development of a modern major transport aeroplane requires an investment of at

The triple-hulled *Aereon III.*

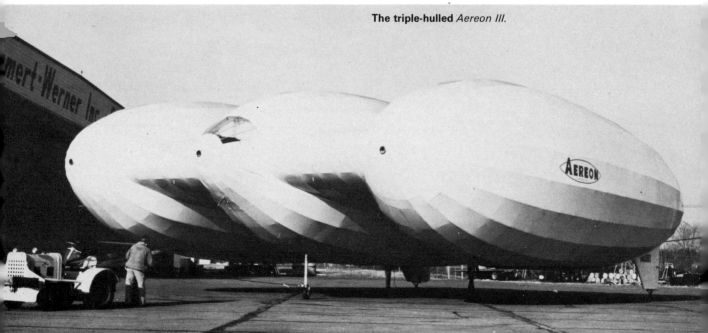

least £500 million). Transport aircraft programmes are often either or entirely government-funded or, as in the case of some of the major civil programmes, indirectly supported by large parallel military programmes paid for by governments. It seems likely therefore that a new large transport airship could only be developed today in a major government programme. Many pressure airship designers do not however see their work as a lead-in to rigids, but as the early stages in the development of even larger pressure ships.

The much more modest undertaking of developing small pressure airships is a different proposition, not only in the technologies involved, but also because smaller resources are required. This should therefore be within reach of relatively small, privately funded organisations.

Hybrid airships, combining features of airships with those of fixed-wing aircraft or helicopters, have been proposed. Another form of hybrid uses both hot air and helium as lifting agents. In large sizes, suitable for heavy-lift or transport purposes, such craft would require a high degree of research and development, especially in the new areas of technology. It therefore seems likely that the cost and difficulty of such developments would approximate more to those of large rigids than to those of small blimps.

Goodyear keeps the flame burning

The US Navy stopped its lighter-than-air activities in 1962. Since then the only practical use of airships has been in advertising and joyriding with small blimps. By far the most prominent in this activity had been the American Goodyear Company, which has built and operated a series of such airships, the *Europa* being the best known in Europe. The *Enterprise*, constructed during 1979, is typical, with a gross volume of 5,740m³ (202,700ft³).

While Goodyear has been the most active manufacturer and operator and the only one to remain continuously in the field, there have been a number of other

Airship Developments AD-500.

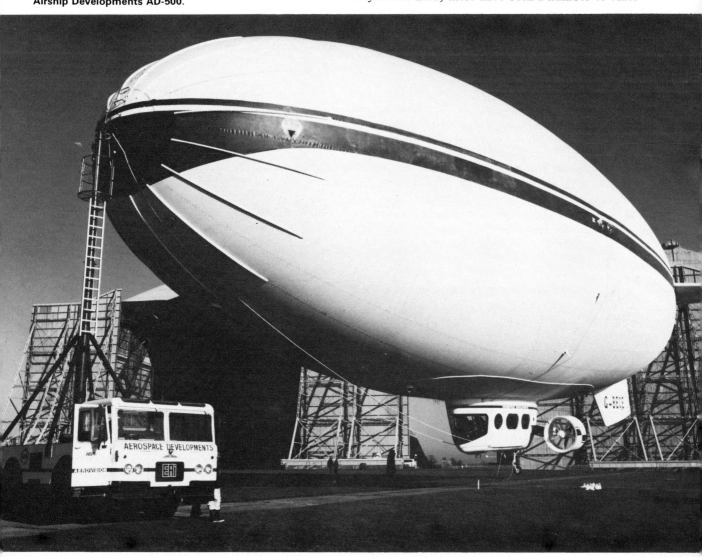

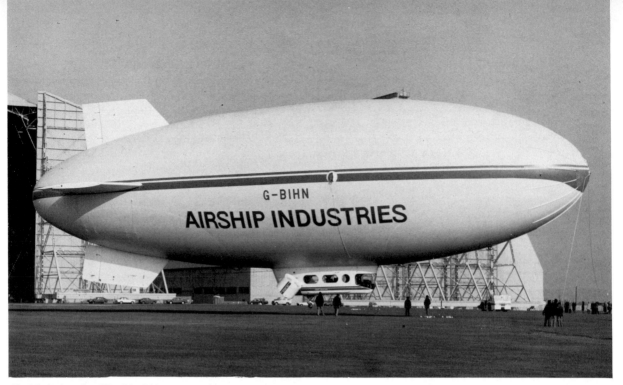

Airship Industries Skyship 500.

organisations which have manufactured or operated similar small ships at various times over the last twenty years. These have included AVO GmbH in West Germany, which from the late 1950s operated an ex-US Navy Goodyear airship, providing advertising for several customers. In 1958 this airship (known as the *Schwab*) was fitted with a new envelope manufactured by Ballonfabrik Augsburg, a company which had first been involved in airship manufacture 60 years earlier.

Ballonfabrik Augsburg made a similar envelope for another West German craft, the *Trumpf*, which was also used for advertising. *Trumpf* continued to fly through the 1960s for various owners. *Schwab* was sold to Japan in the late 1960s but apparently did not do much flying there. The Soviet Union was reported to have flown a small airship, the *Bimbat*, over Moscow in 1965.

The next airship activity of any significance again occurred in West Germany. In 1969 Teodor Wullenkemper founded the WDL airship works in Mulheim. This company had ambitious plans for a whole range of pressure airships, the largest with no less than 64,000m³ (2,260,140ft³) capacity and a maximum gross weight of about 56,700kg (125,000lb). In the event, only two WDL airships of the first and smallest type (about 6,000m³; 212,000ft³) were built and operated over the following three years. A third WDL airship was reported to have been built and flown in Africa in 1976.

Goodyear's European operation
An interesting development in 1972 was the decision by Goodyear to base one of its airships in Europe. This craft was assembled at Cardington and has continued to operate over Europe each summer for the past ten

years. The late 1960s and early 1970s saw a gradual revival of interest in airships in Britain. This attracted a good deal of attention in the press and resulted in Anthony Smith's small blimps *Chitty Bang Bang* (963m³; 34,000ft³) and *Santos Dumont* (934.5m³; 33,000ft³), first flown in 1967 and 1974 respectively, and Aerospace Developments' AD-500 (5,130m³; 181,160ft³), designed by Roger Munk and first flown in 1979. A development of the latter, the Skyship 500, is mentioned later. Meanwhile, in Australia, the small (634m³; 22,385ft³) Mantainer MA-1 *Ardath* was flown in 1978, and other small airships have appeared in Japan, the USA and elsewhere.

Developed in parallel with these pressure airships have been a number of hot-air airships flown in the United Kingdom, Switzerland and the United States. These are intended for advertising but have an impractically low performance for operation in all but the calmest weather, and a very small disposable load.

During the past twenty years there have also been several projects for semi-rigid and even rigid airships which have reached the building stage, although apparently none has flown.

Aereon III, a small experimental triple-hull rigid airship, was built but not flown in the United States in the mid-1960s. Another, in the mid-1970s, was the *Conrad*, reported to be under construction in Arizona. Started at about the same time was the small Tucker TX-1 Silver Hawk, a 651m³ (23,000ft³) semi-rigid that has recently been completed in the United States.

There have been many other proposals for airships, including a small number for very large rigids. It has been said that large rigids are the only types likely to be practical for serious transport purposes, although none has yet got beyond the design stage. This is not so. In Britain there is an organisation with ambitious plans for the development of airships suited to transport roles. Airship Industries was formed in mid-1980 from Thermo-Skyships Ltd and Airship Developments, and in the following year produced a 5,131m³ (181,160ft³) non-rigid airship known as the Skyship 500. This was first flown on September 28, 1981, and is currently undergoing trials. The 50m (164ft 0½in) long envelope is manufactured from a single-ply polyester fabric developed by Airship Industries, and is coated with titanium dioxide polyurethane sealant to minimise loss of helium lifting gas. The nose structure consists of a domed disc formed from Kevlar and carrying the mooring fittings. Two large ballonets are installed fore and aft so that differential inflation can provide some degree of trim. Powerplant comprises two 149kW (200hp) Porsche engines, each driving a ducted propulsor that can be rotated about its pylon to allow vectored thrust for improved performance, manoeuvrability and Vtol capability.

Van Dusen Commercial Development (Canada) Ltd LTA 20-1.

Lighter-than-air cargo-carriers

Derived from the Airship Developments AD-500, the Skyship 500 was proposed to the navies of several countries. It has been suggested that it might be used for maritime patrol, fishery protection and anti-submarine applications. It also gave a clear indication of the suitability of non-rigids as cargo carriers. As a result, Airship Industries is currently manufacturing the follow-on and larger Skyship 600. On the drawing board is the Skyship 5000, which will be a non-rigid with a payload of about 30 tons. A military Skyship 5000 could perform Awacs duties while a commercial version could carry nearly 100 passengers on each of two decks. Continuing work with non-rigids is thought likely to allow for the design of a craft with a 50 to 60-ton payload.

Goodyear in the USA has undertaken a number of feasibility studies of heavy-lift airships, including hybrid types combining the characteristics of airship and helicopter or airship and aeroplane. It may be that one or more of these proposals will lead ultimately to large transport airships, although the very high cost of

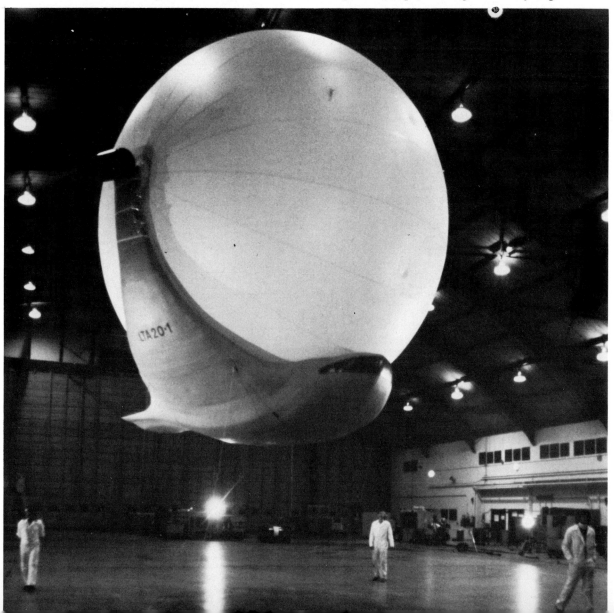

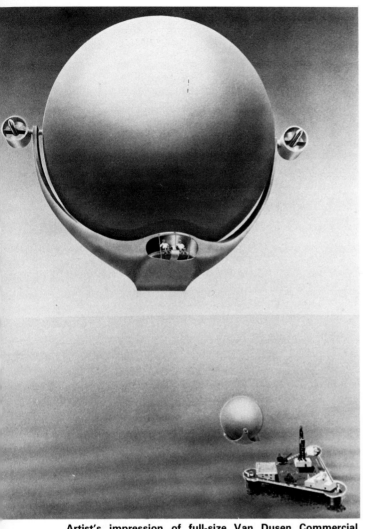

Artist's impression of full-size Van Dusen Commercial Development (Canada) Ltd airships working in support of oil exploration.

60 years of development such aircraft have, despite remarkable reductions in operating costs and the advantage of cross-subsidisation from a rapidly growing passenger transport business, had a hard time establishing themselves as cargo carriers in competition with surface transport. Airships would probably have to do without the benefit of a large passenger operation, a role for which most analysts believe airships are not particularly suitable. For crane and other heavy-lift applications, transport to oil rigs, air/sea rescue and similar suggested roles airships would have to replace helicopters, and the economic advantages would be difficult to evaluate.

Even if the case for airships is accepted and a decision taken to start a new lighter-than-air programme on a reasonable scale, large initial investment would be required for the development and trial operation of several large airships over a protracted period to establish whether they could prove safe, practical, fuel-efficient all-weather craft with operating costs low enough to permit competition with other systems.

Despite some recent interest in airships from a few institutional investors, there is no evidence that private investment on anything like the scale required will be forthcoming immediately. Government funding therefore seems to be essential, although there is as yet no sign that it might become available. However, there are still many people who believe in airships. In Canada Van Dusen Commercial Development (Canada) Ltd has designed airships with unique spherical envelopes to get over many of the recognised problems, while the sphere itself has been designed to rotate to generate additional lift. A radio-controlled scale model designated LTA 20-1 has flown, and design of the full-size LTA 20-01 commercial version has also begun. The LTA 20-01 is expected to have a volume of 118,613m^3 (4,188,790ft^3), a nominal payload of 54,431kg (120,000lb), a cruising speed of 97km/hr (60mph) and a range with maximum payload of 804km (500 miles).

The Soviet Union has also been active in the airship field, having completed trials of a $^{1}/_{10}$th-scale model and being expected to fly a new full-size airship in 1982. This reportedly has a lifting capacity of eight tonnes. An airship of twice this size is also planned, as are others.

development would almost certainly require government funding, of which there is little sign at present.

The majority of those advocating large transport airships see them primarily as cargo carriers, hence the interest of companies such as Federal Express. Their success in this role would however depend on achieving operating costs per ton-mile substantially lower than those of large fixed-wing aeroplanes. Over more than

New Aircraft of The Year

MICHAEL J. H. TAYLOR

Many new aircraft made their first flights during the twelve-month period from June 1981. *New Aircraft of the Year* covers the more important and interesting aircraft in chronological order, with data presented in a style like that of *Jane's All the World's Aircraft*.

Shorts 360 (UK)
36-passenger commuter transport
First flight: June 1, 1981

The Shorts 360 is a stretched development of the Model 330, seating six more passengers in a lengthened fuselage and having strengthened outer wing panels and bracing struts, a new single-fin tail unit, and two 965kW (1,294shp) Pratt & Whitney Aircraft of Canada PT6A-65R turboprops.

Designed specifically for short-haul airline operations over typical commuter stage lengths of about 104nm (193km; 120 miles), the Model 360 is unpress-urised. Passenger features include "walkabout" headroom, air conditioning and other amenities, and more than 0.20m³ (7ft³) of baggage space each.

The first operator to choose the type was Suburban Airlines of Reading, Pennsylvania, which ordered four. Other operators have since placed firm orders or options.

Powerplant: Initially two Pratt & Whitney Aircraft of Canada PT6A-45 turboprops, ultimately two 965kW (1,294shp) PT6A-65R turboprops
Wing span: 22.76m (74ft 8in)
Length overall: 21.49m (70ft 6in)
Typical operating weight empty: 7,480kg (16,490lb)
Max payload (36 passengers): 3,102kg (6,840lb)
Cruising speed at max recommended cruise power: 211kt (391km/hr; 243mph)
Range at 3,050m (10,000ft), cruising at 211kt, ISA, with reserves, 36 passengers: 230nm (425km; 265 miles)
Range, conditions as above, with max fuel: 570nm (1,055km; 655 miles)

Shorts 360. *(Shorts)*

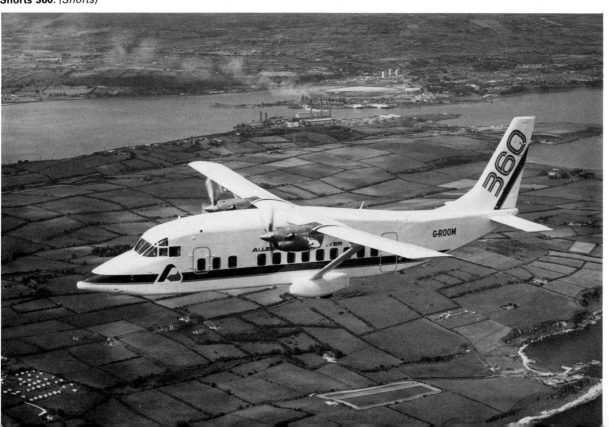

Tesori Scale Reggiane 2000 (Canada)
Three-quarter-scale representation of Reggiane 2000
Falco I fighter of 1938
First flight: June 1, 1981

Robert Tesori designed and built this scale representation of the Italian Reggiane Falco I single-seat fighter using information gleaned from a small plastic model kit. It first flew from Edmonton International Airport in mid-1981.

To allow an early first flight Mr Tesori fitted the representation with the modified plywood-covered wooden wings of his Piel Emeraude, and a hydraulically actuated retractable landing gear. Aluminium alloy wings and a modified Globe Swift landing gear are to be retrofitted. The fuselage is made of aluminium alloy with stressed skins.

Powerplant: One 149kW (200hp) Avco Lycoming IO-360-A1A
Weight empty: 572kg (1,260lb)
Max T-O weight: 884kg (1,950lb)
Max level speed at S/L: 152kt (282km/hr; 175mph)
Max cruising speed: 143kt (266km/hr; 165mph)
Max rate of climb at S/L: 305m (1,000ft)/min

Whatley Special (USA)
Homebuilt single-seat light biplane
First flight: June 23, 1981

Originally known as the Econobipe because of its low operating cost, the Special was designed and built by Vascoe Whatley Jr. Based partly on the Gere Sport of the 1930s, it is said to be easy to build and fly. The airframe is made mainly of wood.

Powerplant: One 2,232cc Volkswagen modified car engine
Wing span, upper: 6.22m (20ft 5in)
Wing span, lower: 5.82m (19ft 1in)
Weight empty: 222kg (490lb)
Max T-O weight: 336kg (740lb)
Cruising speed: 65kt (121km/hr; 75mph)

Goldwing Gold Duster (USA)
Single-seat agricultural microlight
First flight: 1981

The Gold Duster, a new version of the Goldwing, was unveiled in 1981 at the National Agricultural Aviation Association in Las Vegas. By January 1982 two prototypes had been completed and production was starting, the aircraft being available in ready-to-fly or kit form.

The Gold Duster is basically a Goldwing with structural modifications to permit the useful load to be increased to 159kg (350lb). A 57lit (15 US gal) hopper and two Micronair mini-atomisers are fitted, together with variable restrictors, gate valves, a fan-driven pump, and an optional flowmeter. Fitted with this ultra-low-volume (ULV) system, the Gold Duster has a typical operating speed of 52kt (97km/hr; 60mph) and can cover a swath of 12m (40ft). It can dispense 0.48-3.8lit (1 US pint to 1 US gal) per minute from each spray head. Fuel capacity is reduced to 9.5lit (2.5 US gal). The UK (Euro Wing) version has a British dispersal system.

Powerplant: One 22.4kW (30hp) Cuyuna 430D two-cylinder two-stroke
Wing span: 9.14m (30ft 0in)
Length overall: 3.66m (12ft 0in)
Weight empty: 118kg (260lb)
Max T-O weight: 286kg (630lb)
Max level speed: 61kt (112km/hr; 70mph)
Max cruising speed: 52kt (97km/hr; 60mph)
Econ cruising speed: 43.5kt (80km/hr; 50mph)
Max rate of climb at S/L: 183m (600ft)/min
Service ceiling: 4,265m (14,000ft)
Range with max fuel: 65nm (120km; 75 miles)
Endurance: 1hr 15min

Smith AJ-2 (USA)
Homebuilt two-seat monoplane
First flight: July 15, 1981

The work of former gliding champion A. J. Smith, the design of this tandem two-seat monoplane embodies a high degree of sailplane technology. The aircraft was built mainly by Leonard Niemi, making extensive use of glassfibre.

Intended originally for touring and cross-country flights, with the forward seat doubling as extra baggage space when not occupied, the AJ-2 has competed in the LBF efficiency race.

Smith AJ-2.

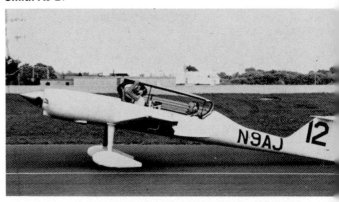

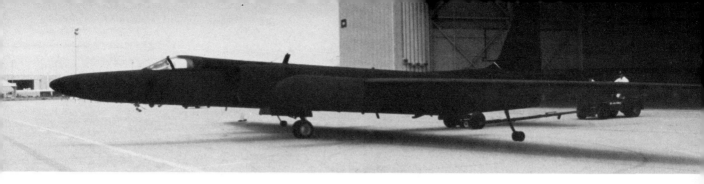

Lockheed TR-1A. *(USAF)*

Powerplant: One 160kW (215hp) Avco Lycoming
IO-360-A1B6 flat-four
Wing span: 7.31m (24ft 0in)
Length overall: 6.70m (22ft 0in)
Weight empty: 500kg (1,102lb)
Max T-O weight: 771kg (1,700lb)
Max level speed: 259kt (480km/hr; 298mph)
Max cruising speed (75% power): 248kt (460km/hr;
   285mph)

Turner T-77 (T-40C) (USA)
Two-seat sporting monoplane
First flight: July 16, 1981

The T-77 utilises the Turner T-40A fuselage and
incorporates simplified model-aeroplane-type construction. The wing is based on a highly modified and
computer-developed version of the Nasa GAW
general-aviation section and incorporates a quick-
folding mechanism. Aerodynamically operated
leading-edge slats, manually operated full-span split
flaps, spoilers without supplemental ailerons (in six
sections, for roll control), and ground spoilers are fitted
to the wings. The airframe is of wooden construction,
with a fir structure covered by mahogany plywood.

Powerplant: One 112kW (150hp) Avco Lycoming flat-
   four
Wing span: 8.53m (28ft 0in)
Length overall: 6.12m (20ft 1in)
Weight empty: 376kg (828lb)
Max T-O weight: 748kg (1,650lb)
Max level speed at S/L: 165kt (306km/hr; 190mph)
Max cruising speed: 152kt (282km/hr; 175mph)
Max rate of climb at S/L: 457m (1,500ft)/min
Estimated service ceiling: 6,400m (21,000ft)
Range with max payload, 20min reserves: 521nm
   (965km; 600 miles)

Lockheed TR-1A (USA)
High-altitude reconnaissance aircraft
First flight: August 1, 1981

The TR-1A single-seat tactical reconnaissance aircraft
is based on the U-2. Tooling for the latter had been kept
in store, allowing the production line to be reopened in

FY 1980. Described by the Department of Defense as
"equipped with a variety of electronic sensors to provide continuously available, day or night, high-altitude
all-weather stand-off surveillance of the battle area in
direct support of the US and Allied ground and air
forces during peace, crisis, and war situations," the
TR-1A carries an advanced synthetic-aperture radar
system (ASARS) in the form of a UPD-X sideways-
looking airborne radar (SLAR), and modern electronic
countermeasures (ECM). Seen as a replacement for the
abandoned Compass Cope RPV, the TR-1 is intended
primarily for use in Europe, where the SLAR will be
able to see approximately 30nm (55km; 35 miles) into
hostile territory from outside the actual or potential
battle area. The total USAF requirement is for 35
aircraft, all TR-1As except for two two-seat TR-1Bs.

Powerplant: One 75.6kN (17,000lb st) Pratt & Whitney
   J75-P-13B turbojet
Wing span: 31.39m (103ft 0in)
Length overall: 19.20m (63ft 0in)
Max T-O weight: 18,143kg (40,000lb)
Max cruising speed at over 21,650m (70,000ft): more
   than 373kt (692km/hr; 430mph)
Operational ceiling: 27,430m (90,000ft)
Max range: more than 2,605nm (4,830km; 3,000 miles)
Endurance: 12hr

Southern Aero Sports Scorpion (UK)
Single or two-seat microlight
First flight: August 1981

The Scorpion entered production in 1981 and by the
end of that year more than 100 had been ordered by
customers in Saudi Arabia, South Africa, Sweden and
the UK. A two-seat version was expected to become
available in 1982.
   The aircraft itself has marked wing dihedral, three-
axis control ("spoilerons," elevators and rudder), and
double-surface Dacron-covered wings.

Powerplant: One 40.25kW (54hp) Fuji Robin two-
   cylinder two-stroke is typical, but other engines are
   available
Weight empty: approx 84kg (185lb)
Max level speed: approx 69.5kt (129km/hr; 80mph)
Max rate of climb at S/L: 305m (1,000ft)/min

Mortensen/Rutan Amsoil Racer (USA)
Single-seat racing biplane
First flight: August 1981

Dan Mortensen has built and flown a biplane racer designed at his request by Burt Rutan. Construction began in January 1981 and by the end of September the aircraft had accumulated 17hr in the air.

The illustration of the Racer that appears with *Strange Wings, Strange Things* (see page 43) shows it to be similar in configuration to the Quickie, but with several important differences. Built of foam, glassfibre and graphite, it has non-structural I-type struts between the foreplanes and rear wings, and a T-tail.

Powerplant: One 119kW (160hp) Avco Lycoming
      IO-320
Wing span: 6.71m (22ft 0in)
Length overall: 6.10m (20ft 0in)
Weight empty: 386kg (850lb)
Max T-O weight: 510kg (1,125lb)
Recorded level speed: 201kt (373km/hr; 232 mph)

McDonnell Douglas DC-8 Super 71 (USA)
Long-range airliner
First flight: August 15, 1981

By replacing the existing engines in the DC-8 Srs 61, 62 and 63 with General Electric/Snecma CFM56 or Pratt & Whitney JT8D-209 turbofans McDonnell Douglas is producing the new Super 71, 72 and 73 respectively. The first such modification resulted in a Super 71 in August 1981, at which time conversion of the first Super 72 and 73 was well advanced. Deliveries of the Super 71 began in April 1982, to Delta and United.

McDonnell Douglas expects the Super 71, 72 and 73 with CFM56-2-1C engines to be the world's quietest large four-engined transports when they enter service.

McDonnell Douglas DC-8 Super 71.

The new engines offer improved performance, including reduced take-off run, increased range, and fuel savings over a 3,000nm (5,560km; 3,455-mile) route of as much as 7,711kg (17,000lb) for the DC-8 Super 71.

Powerplant: As above
Wing span: 45.23m (148ft 5in)
Length overall: 57.12m (187ft 5in)
Operating weight empty: 73,800kg (162,700lb)
Max payload: 30,240kg (66,665lb)
Max T-O weight: 147,415kg (325,000lb)
Max level speed: 521kt (965km/hr; 600mph)
Cruising speed: Mach 0.80

BAe 146 (UK)
Short-range transport
First flight: September 3, 1981

In July 1978 British Aerospace finally went ahead with production of the BAe 146 following several years of design and development work. Basic design aims were: passenger seating standards comparable with those of current wide-bodied transports, competitive operating costs, good airfield performance and low noise levels.

The BAe 146 Series 100, rolled out on May 20, 1981, is designed to operate from short semi-prepared airstrips with minimal ground facilities, and to seat 71-93. A mixed passenger/freight version is planned. The 82-109-seat Series 200 will operate from paved runways only, and has a longer fuselage, increased max T-O weight, increased underfloor cargo volume and greater range; maximum operating speed is slightly reduced. Initial deliveries of production Series 100s were scheduled for September/October 1982.

The following details apply to the 146 Series 100.

Powerplant: Four Avco Lycoming ALF502 R-3 turbofans, each rated at 29.8kN (6,700lb st)
Wing span: 26.34m (86ft 5in)

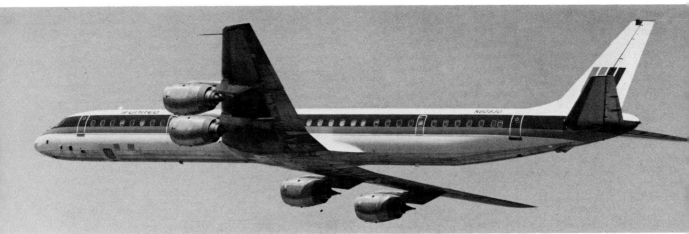

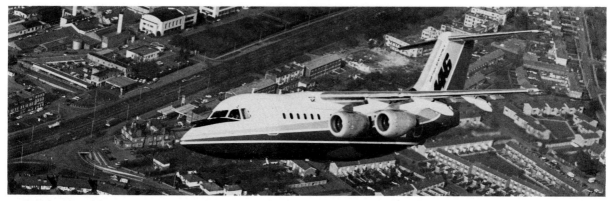

BAe 146 Series 100. *(BAe)*

Length overall: 26.16m (85ft 10in)
Typical operating weight empty: 20,670kg (45,570lb)
Max payload: 8,020kg (17,680lb)
Max T-O weight: 33,840-36,628kg (74,600-80,750lb)
Max operating speed: Mach 0.70
Max cruising speed at 7,925m (26,000ft): 419kt
(776km/hr; 482mph)
Econ cruising speed at 9,145m (30,000ft): 371kt
(687km/hr; 427mph)
*Range with max fuel, incl 293kg (645lb) fuel for ground
and airborne manoeuvres, plus reserves:* 1,550nm
(2,872km; 1,785 miles)
Range with max payload, allowances as above: 510nm
(945km; 587 miles)

MBA Mistral Trainer (UK)
Training, cropspraying, aerial photography and
reconnaissance microlight
First flight: September 22, 1981

The two-seat Mistral Trainer prototype was constructed by MBA (Micro Biplane Aviation) with assistance from personnel at British Aerospace and Rolls-
Royce Filton. A single-seat cropspraying version of the
aircraft, with a Micronair dispersal system installed
behind the pilot's seat, was flown in January 1982, by
which time ten Trainers had been sold.
The following details refer to the two-seat Trainer.

Powerplant: One 22.4kW (30hp) Cuyuna 430R two-
cylinder two-stroke
Wing span: 12.19m (40ft 0in)
Length overall: 3.73m (12ft 3in)
Weight empty: 127kg (280lb)
Max T-O weight: 317.5kg (700lb)
Max level and cruising speed: 42kt (77km/hr; 48mph)
Econ cruising speed: 33kt (61km/hr; 38mph)
Max rate of climb at S/L: 122m (400ft)/min
Service ceiling (estimated): 1,525m (5,000ft)
Range with standard fuel: 87nm (161km; 100 miles)
Endurance: 3hr

Sikorsky YEH-60A Black Hawk (USA)
Communications jamming helicopter
First flight: September 24, 1981

In September 1981 Sikorsky produced the first YEH-
60A, the pre-production prototype of an ECM variant
of the Black Hawk. Designed to intercept and jam
enemy communications, the EH-60A embodies Quick
Fix II, 816kg (1,800lb) of electronics equipment
including four dipole antennae mounted on the rear
fuselage and a deployable whip antenna beneath the
fuselage. The EH-60A Quick Fix II represents but one
component of the US Army's Special Electronic Mission Aircraft (SEMA) programme. The Army plans to
acquire 77 EH-60As.
The following details refer to the UH-60A Black
Hawk.

Powerplant: Two 1,151kW (1,560shp) General Electric
T700-GE-700 advanced-technology turboshafts
Main-rotor diameter: 16.36m (53ft 8in)
Length of fuselage: 15.26m (50ft 0¾in)
Weight empty: 4,819kg (10,624lb)
Max T-O weight: 9,185kg (20,250lb)
Max level speed at S/L: 160kt (296km/hr; 184mph)
Max level speed at max T-O weight: 158kt (293km/hr;
182mph)
Max cruising speed: 145kt (269km/hr; 167mph)
Service ceiling: 5,790m (19,000ft)
Range at max T-O weight, 30min reserves: 324nm
(600km; 373 miles)
Endurance: 2hr 18min

Piper (PA-31-350) T-1020 (USA)
Eleven-seat commuter airliner
First flight: September 25, 1981

Based on the PA-31-350 Chieftain, the T-1020 retains
the same basic airframe and is powered by two 261kW
(350hp) Avco Lycoming TIO-540 flat-six turbocharged engines; for this application the TIO-540
has been cleared for a special commuter time between
overhauls (TBO) of 1,800hr. The main changes affect

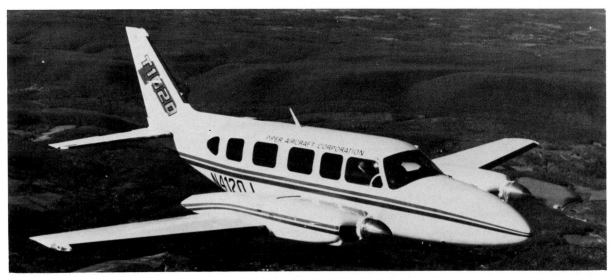

Piper T-1020.

the interior, which has been "hardened" to airline standards to accommodate a crew of two and nine passengers. The doors and landing gear have been strengthened to withstand the high-frequency short-haul operations of a commuter line. Most of the 317kg (700lb) of baggage can be stored outside the cabin.

Design of the T-1020 began at the end of April 1981 and construction of a prototype started the following August. Delivery of production aircraft will take place immediately after certification.

Powerplant: As above
Wing span: 12.40m (40ft 8in)
Length overall: 10.55m (34ft 7½in)
Weight empty: 2,018kg (4,450lb)
Max payload: 1,157kg (2,550lb)
Max T-O weight: 3,175kg (7,000lb)
Max level speed at 3,050m (10,000ft): 231kt (428km/hr; 266mph)
Max cruising speed at 3,050m (10,000ft): 221kt (410km/hr; 254mph)
Econ cruising speed at 3,050m (10,000ft): 210kt (389km/hr; 242mph)
Max rate of climb at S/L: 341m (1,120ft)/min
Service ceiling: 7,315m (24,000ft)
Range: 480nm (890km; 553 miles)

Boeing 767 (USA)
Medium-range airliner
First flight: September 26, 1981

Having received an order from United Airlines for 30 Model 767s, Boeing announced in July 1978 its intention of launching full-scale development of this airliner. A year later work began on the first Model 767, with a completely new fuselage 1.24m (4ft 1in) wider than that of the Model 757 to allow a two-aisle seating arrangement. The basic model is the 767-200 accommodating 211 passengers. The first Model 767 was rolled out on August 4, 1981, and flew during the following month. Deliveries to United were expected to begin in August 1982. It is also intended to market a

Boeing Model 767. *(Boeing)*

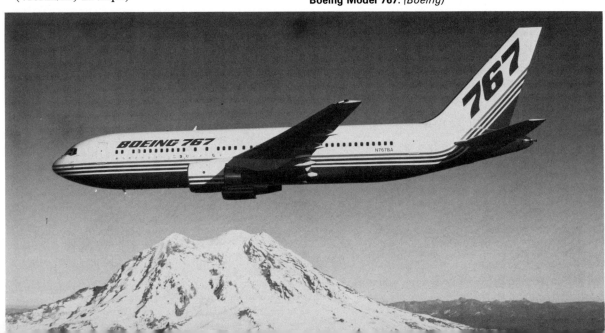

medium-range version with reduced fuel capacity, and a variant with a higher gross weight. Two-crew flight decks will be standard from the start.

A total of 173 Model 767s had been ordered by March 1982, with a further 138 on option. Biggest customer United currently has 39 on order, followed by American Airlines with 30. The largest number ordered by a non-American airline is the 25 for All Nippon (Japan). Important manufacturing subcontracts have been awarded by Boeing to Grumman, Vought, Canadair, Aeritalia and three Japanese companies.

Powerplant: Two 212.6kN (47,800lb st) Pratt & Whitney JT9D-7R4D or two 213kN (47,900lb st) General Electric CF6-80A high-bypass turbofans. Rolls-Royce RB.211s are being studied
Accommodation: 211 passengers basic. Alternative single-class layouts for 230, 242 or 255 tourist-class passengers, or a maximum seating capacity of 289
Wing span: 47.57m (156ft 1in)
Length overall: 48.51m (159ft 2in)
Weight empty (767-200 with JT9D-7R4Ds): 74,548kg (164,352lb)
Max T-O weight (model and engines as above): 136,080kg (300,000lb)
Normal cruising speed: Mach 0.80
Service ceiling (model and engines as above): 11,885m (39,000ft)
Design range (model and engines as above): 2,780nm (5,152km; 3,201 miles)

Zlin 526 AFM Condor (Czechoslovakia)
Trainer
First flight: Autumn 1981?

The Condor is a further aircraft in the successful Zlin 126/226/326/526/726 series, combining the fuselage of the Z 526 AFS Akrobat (lengthened by approximately 0.20m; 8in) with a slightly extended version of the wing fitted to the Z 326; the new wing also carries tip tanks. The engine drives an Avia V410 two-blade propeller.

Powerplant: One 157kW (210hp) Avia M 337 inverted six-cylinder air-cooled inline
Wing span over tip tanks: 10.59m (34ft 9in)
Length overall: 8.00m (26ft 3in)
Weight empty: 680kg (1,499lb)
Max T-O weight: 910kg (2,006lb)
Max level speed: 142kt (263km/hr; 163mph) IAS
Max cruising speed: 120kt (222km/hr; 138mph) IAS
Range with max fuel: 485nm (900km; 559 miles)
Endurance at cruising speed: 3hr 50min

Schweizer Ag-Cat B-Plus (USA)
Agricultural aircraft
Resumed production: October 1981

The original Ag-Cat agricultural biplane flew for the first time in May 1957. Deliveries began in 1959 and approximately 2,455 Ag-Cats were built by Schweizer under sub-contract from Grumman/Gulfstream American over the next twenty years. In October 1981 production of the Ag-Cat resumed with the improved Ag-Cat B-Plus following Schweizer's purchase of the rights in the aircraft, of which two versions are being offered. The first is the B-Plus/600 (G-164B), powered by a 447.5kW (600hp) Pratt & Whitney R-1340 radial and with other improvements including a hopper with 40 per cent greater capacity. The other is the B-Plus/450 (G-164B), generally similar to the B-Plus/600 but powered by a 335.5kW (450hp) Pratt & Whitney R-985 radial.

McDonnell Douglas AV-8B Harrier II (USA)
V/Stol combat aircraft
First flight (development aircraft): November 5, 1981

The AV-8B Harrier II programme calls for the development of an advanced V/Stol attack aircraft which, without too much departure from the existing Harrier airframe, will be capable of virtually double the aircraft's existing weapons load/combat radius. As a

McDonnell Douglas AV-8B Harrier II. *(McDonnell Douglas)*

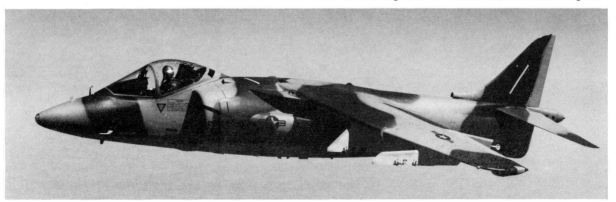

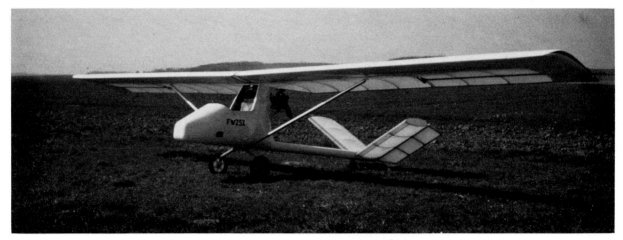

Aerostructure Pipistrelle 2B.

first stage in the programme, McDonnell Douglas and the USMC modified two AV-8As as prototype YAV-8Bs. The first of these flew on November 9, 1978. Aerodynamic changes include the use of a supercritical wing, the addition of under-gun-pod strakes and a retractable dam forward of the pods (to increase lift for vertical take-off), larger wing trailing-edge flaps and drooped ailerons, and redesigned engine air intakes. The leading-edge root extensions (LERX) developed originally by British Aerospace for the UK-designed Big Wing Harrier will also be standard.

The first of four full-scale development aircraft was flown in November 1981. Navy Bureau of Inspection and Survey trials are planned for late 1983, leading to a light attack squadron operational readiness date of mid-1985. The USMC has a stated requirement for 336 AV-8Bs. The FY 1982 defence budget allows for an initial twelve Harrier IIs. The RAF is also to receive Harrier IIs, as GR5s, for service from 1986. Final assembly of the RAF aircraft and manufacture of approximately 40 per cent of Harrier II components will be undertaken by BAe. On the engines, 75 per cent of the work for the USMC will be carried out by Rolls-Royce, and 25 per cent by Pratt & Whitney.

Powerplant: One Rolls-Royce Pegasus 11-21E (F402-RR-406) vectored-thrust turbofan rated at 95.64kN (21,150lb st)
Wing span: 9.25m (30ft 4in)
Length overall: 14.12m (46ft 4in)
Basic operating weight empty: 5,783kg (12,750lb)
Max external stores: 4,173kg (9,200lb)
Max T-O weight (STO): 13,494kg (29,750lb)
Max Mach number in level flight at altitude: Mach 0.91
Max level speed at S/L: 585kt (1,083km/hr; 673mph)
Operational radius with short T-O, carrying seven Mk 82 Snakeye bombs, external fuel tanks, no loiter: more than 650nm (1,204km; 748 miles)
Operational radius with short T-O, carrying twelve Snakeye bombs, internal fuel, 1hr loiter: more than 150nm (278km; 172 miles)

Aerostructure Pipistrelle 2B (France)
Single-seat microlight monoplane
First flight: Late 1981

The Pipistrelle 2B is a single-seat open-cockpit aircraft with a strut-braced, high-mounted, rigid but foldable wing, a V-tail and an engine driving a pusher propeller. It was designed and built by a group of enthusiasts who, after visiting the Paris Salon, decided to make their own microlight. Design took approximately two months and construction three. By July 1982 a further ten aircraft had been built and sold.

Powerplant: One JPX PUL 425 engine
Wing span: 11.2m (36ft 9in)
Weight empty: 110kg (243lb)
Max T-O weight: 202kg (445lb)
Max level speed: 70kt (130km/hr; 81mph)
Max cruising speed: 54kt (100km/hr; 62mph)
Econ cruising speed: 46kt (85km/hr; 53mph)
Max rate of climb at S/L: 120m (395ft)/min
Service ceiling: 3,000m (9,440ft)
Range: 162nm (300km; 186 miles)
Endurance with max fuel: 3hr

OMAC I (USA)
Light business aircraft
First flight: December 11, 1981

OMAC (Old Man's Aircraft Company) was founded to develop and market a low-cost, high-performance, economical six/eight-seat turboprop-powered business aircraft. The resulting OMAC I is of canard configuration, with high-mounted mainplane and a low-set foreplane. OMAC will produce the light alloy wings and semi-monocoque fuselage for production aircraft, the remaining components and assemblies being contracted out. The company will be responsible for final assembly and flight testing.

The prototype OMAC I first flew in late 1981 and was expected to receive certification under FAR Pt 23 in the late summer of 1982. By February 1982 a total of 30 OMAC Is had been ordered.

Powerplant: One 522kW (700shp) Avco Lycoming LTP101-700A-A1 turboprop driving a pusher propeller
Wing span: 10.67m (35ft 0in)
Foreplane span: 5.23m (17ft 2in)
Length overall: 9.14m (30ft 0in)
Weight empty (estimated): 1,451kg (3,200lb)
Max T-O weight (estimated): 2,585kg (5,700lb)
Max level speed (estimated): 260kt (482km/hr; 299mph)
Cruising speed (estimated): 248kt (460km/hr; 286mph)
Econ cruising speed (estimated): 217kt (402km/hr; 250mph)
Max rate of climb at S/L (estimated): 610m (2,000ft)/min
Certificated ceiling (estimated): 7,620m (25,000ft)
Max range at econ cruising speed, with allowances for 1hr hold (estimated): 2,950nm (5,467km; 3,397 miles)

NDN 6 Fieldmaster (UK)
Agricultural aircraft
First flight: December 17, 1981

The Fieldmaster is being developed by NDN, partly financed by the UK National Research Development Corporation. In an entirely new approach to agricultural aircraft design, the Fieldmaster has a titanium chemical hopper which forms an integral part of the fuselage structure, its outer surface being contoured to serve as the skin of that fuselage section. The single 559kW (750shp) Pratt & Whitney Aircraft of Canada PT6A-34AG turboprop is mounted on the front of the hopper, the aft fuselage to its rear, and the wings are built directly on to each side of the hopper's base. The cockpit can accommodate a second seat in tandem if required. Removable dual controls are standard, simplifying flight training and check-out procedures.

The Fieldmaster's wings are fitted with full-span auxiliary trailing-edge flaps which embody a liquid spray dispersal system that discharges directly into the downwash of the flaps, so ensuring the best possible crop penetration. Hopper capacity is 1,996kg (4,400lb) of dry or 2,642lit (581 Imp gal) of liquid chemical.

Powerplant: As above
Wing span: 15.32m (50ft 3in)
Length overall: 11.02m (36ft 2in)
Max level speed, clean: 142kt (263km/hr; 164mph)
Empty weight: 1,973kg (4,350lb)
Max payload: 2,563kg (5,650lb)
Max T-O weight: 4,536kg (10,000lb)
Cruising speed (75% power): 135kt (249km/hr; 155mph)
Range: 1,020nm (1,889km; 1,174 miles)

NDN 6 Fieldmaster.

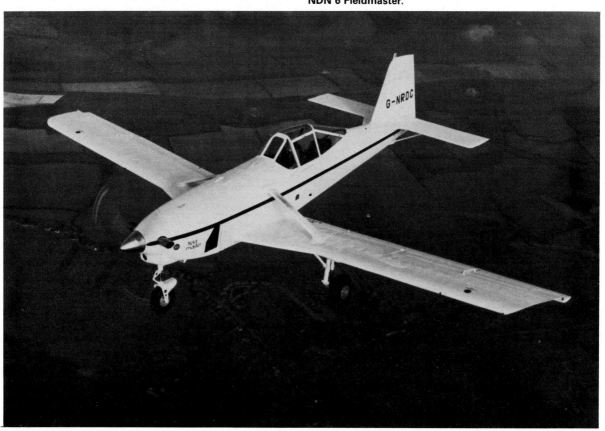

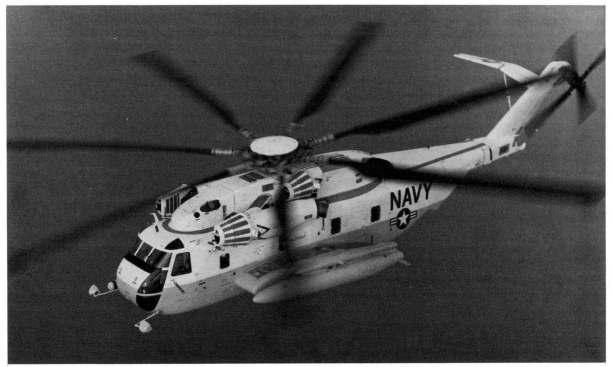

Sikorsky CH/MH-53E.

Kelly-D (USA)
Homebuilt two-seat biplane
First flight: December 20, 1981

The Kelly-D tandem two-seat biplane was designed in 1977 by Dudley R. Kelly, who was seeking improved efficiency and easier and cheaper construction by comparison with other designs in the same category. Construction of the prototype, by Jim Foster, began almost two years later.

Powerplant: One 86kW (115hp) Avco Lycoming O-235 flat-four
Wing span: 7.42m (24ft 4in)
Length overall: 5.87m (19ft 3in)
Basic operating weight empty: 352kg (775lb)
Max T-O weight: 635kg (1,400lb)
Max level speed at 1,525m (5,000ft): 91kt (169km/hr; 105mph)
Max cruising speed at 1,525m (5,000ft): 78kt (145km/hr; 90mph)
Max rate of climb at S/L: 229m (750ft)/min
Range with max fuel, 20min reserves: 234nm (435km; 270 miles)

Sikorsky CH/MH-53E (USA)
Minesweeping helicopter
First flight: December 23, 1981

The US Navy's stated requirement for more than 200 Super Stallions included a number of the proposed

MH-53E Airborne Mine Countermeasures (AMCM) helicopters. To evaluate the configuration the first production CH-53E was modified and given the temporary designation CH/MH-53E. Although it was then essentially an AMCM-equipped Super Stallion, actual production MH-53Es could differ by having enlarged sponsons to increase fuel capacity and so allow longer missions. The type could also have a secondary vertical replenishment role.

Following company trials the CH/MH-53E was flown to the US Navy's Coast Systems Center, Panama City, Florida, where dynamic tow testing with mine countermeasures equipment began in early 1982. In April, when the test helicopter was fitted with enlarged sponsons, it was announced that the Department of Defense had awarded Sikorsky a contract to continue research and development work on the MH-53E, including the production of a prototype in operational minesweeping configuration. The first full production MH-53Es could be delivered in late 1986, and initial plans call for a total of 57.

The following details refer to the CH-53E Super Stallion.

Powerplant: Three General Electric T64-GE-416 turboshafts, each with a max rating of 3,266kW (4,380shp) for 10min, intermediate rating of 3,091kW (4,145shp) for 30min, and max continuous rating of 2,756kW (3,696shp)
Main rotor diameter: 24.08m (79ft 0in)
Length of fuselage: 22.35m (73ft 4in)
Weight empty: 15,071kg (33,226lb)
Max T-O weight: 33,339kg (73,500lb)

Max level speed: 170kt (315km/hr; 196mph)
Cruising speed: 150kt (278km/hr; 173mph)
Max rate of climb at S/L: 838m (2,750ft)/min
Service ceiling: 5,640m (18,500ft)
Range, at optimum cruise condition: 1,120nm (2,075km; 1,290 miles)

Fairchild Swearingen Metro IIIA (USA)
19/20-passenger commuter airliner
First flight: December 31, 1981

The Metro IIIA is a version of the Metro III for operators wishing to standardise on a common family of P&WC engines throughout a multi-type fleet of aircraft. The Metro IIIA therefore has the III's Garrett engines replaced by two Pratt & Whitney Aircraft of Canada PT6A-45-6R turboprops, each flat-rated to 820kW (1,100shp). Other changes include new stream-lined nacelles, aluminium clamshell cowlings which open wide for easy access, redesigned landing gear and a new high-volume environmental control system with improved ground air-conditioning capability.

Deliveries of the Metro IIIA to regional airline customers are scheduled to begin in mid-1983.

Powerplant: See above
Wing span: 17.37m (57ft 0in)
Length overall: 18.09m (59ft 4¼in)
Max T-O weight: 6,577kg (14,500lb)
Cruising speed, max landing weight of 6,350kg (14,000lb), at 3,050m (10,000ft): 273kt (506km/hr; 314mph)
Max rate of climb at S/L: 625m (2,050ft)/min
Service ceiling: 8,100m (26,600ft)
Range with max payload, max cruising power at 7,620m (25,000ft): 663nm (1,228km; 763 miles)

Gulfstream Commander Jetprop 900 (USA)
Eight-seat light transport
Introduced: 1982

The Commander Jetprop 900 combines the powerplant of the Jetprop 840 with the airframe of the Jetprop 1000.

Powerplant: Two Garrett TPE331-5-254K turboprops, each flat-rated to a max output of 557.8kW (748shp)
Wing span: 15.89m (52ft 1½in)
Length overall: 13.10m (42ft 11¾in)
Weight empty: 3,174kg (6,998lb)
Max payload: 908kg (2,002lb)
Max T-O weight: 4,853kg (10,700lb)
Max operating speed: 252kt (467km/hr; 290mph) CAS

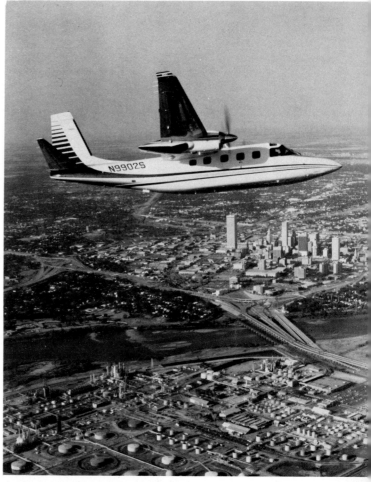

Gulfstream Commander Jetprop 900.

Max cruising speed at 3,050m (10,000ft): 289kt (536km/hr; 333mph)
Econ cruising speed at 10,670m (35,000ft): 251kt (465km/hr; 289mph)
Max rate of climb at S/L: 847m (2,779ft)/min
Service ceiling (max certificated): 10,670m (35,000ft)
Range with max payload at 9,450m (31,000ft), 45min reserves: 915nm (1,695km; 1,053 miles)
Range with max standard fuel, altitude and reserves as above: 1,721nm (3,189km; 1,982 miles)
Range with max optional fuel, altitude and reserves as above: 1,966nm (3,643km; 2,264 miles)

Hawk GafHawk 125 (USA)
Turboprop freighter
First flight: 1982

Having experienced problems in transporting its equipment for oil and water well drilling and fencing, Hawk Industries set about designing an aircraft to suit its own needs. The outcome is the GafHawk 125 (Gaf = general aviation freighter), which was scheduled to make its first flight in early 1982.

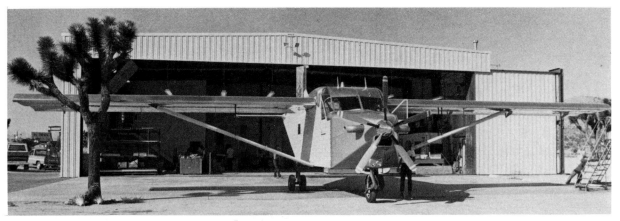

Hawk GafHawk 125.

Prime characteristics of the GafHawk 125 are Stol capability for operation into and from small unprepared strips; a turboprop engine for economic operation; a square-section fuselage for maximum utilisation of internal capacity; under-tail loading of bulk cargo at truckbed height; and a single engine for economy, ease of certification and single-pilot operation. Construction of the prototype was almost complete by the end of 1981.

Powerplant: Prototype has one Pratt & Whitney Aircraft of Canada PT6A-45R turboprop rated at 875kW (1,173shp) standard maximum
Accommodation: Main cabin volume augmented by usable space under flight deck, accommodating pipes and timber up to 6.1m (20ft) in length with rear loading door closed
Wing span: 21.79m (71ft 6in)
Length overall: 14.30m (46ft 11in)
Weight empty: 2,835kg (6,250lb)
Max T-O weight: 5,670kg (12,500lb)
Max cruising speed at 3,050m (10,000ft): 152kt (282km/hr; 175mph)
Econ cruising speed (55% power) at 3,050m (10,000ft): 126kt (233km/hr; 145mph)
Max rate of climb at S/L: 290m (950ft)/min
Service ceiling: 5,485m (18,000ft)
Range with max fuel: 900nm (1,668km; 1,036 miles)

Rutan Model 72 Grizzly (USA)
Proof-of-concept research aircraft
First flight: January 22, 1982

The unusually configured Grizzly was built to investigate the Stol potential of a tandem-wing aircraft, new amphibious floats, and a number of structural concepts.

Rolled out at Mojave Airport on January 14, 1982, it is a four-seater with an airframe made of carbon-fibre and glassfibre composites, together with the foam-core structure that has become a feature of Rutan designs. It

is a canard/tandem-wing aircraft, and the mainplane and canards are linked by fuel-carrying booms. Initial tests are being carried out with a non-retractable tailwheel undercarriage, the curved main gear struts of which each carry dual low-pressure tyres. It is intended ultimately to fit a unique system of floats to give amphibious capability without gear retraction or water rudders.

On January 22, 1982, the Grizzly made a 2hr 36min first flight. No detailed specification and performance figures had been received at the time of writing (see also *Strange Wings, Strange Things,* page 43).

Powerplant: One 134kW (180hp) Avco Lycoming IO-360-B flat-four

Piper PA-28R-300XBT Pillan (USA/Chile)
Two-seat basic/intermediate military trainer
First flight (Chilean-assembled): January 30, 1982

Piper has developed a derivative of the Cherokee series known as the Pillan to meet the requirements of the Chilean Air Force for a new basic/intermediate trainer with full aerobatic capability. The type has two seats in tandem under a one-piece canopy. Following the production of two examples by Piper, an initial batch of three more were supplied to Chile in kit form for final assembly. The first of these flew on January 30, 1982.

Powerplant: One 224kW (300hp) Avco Lycoming AEIO-540 flat-six
Wing span: 8.81m (28ft 11in)
Length overall: 7.97m (26ft 1¾in)
Max level speed at 1,315kg (2,900lb) AUW: 173kt (321km/hr; 199mph)
Cruising speed (75% power), AUW as above: 166kt (308km/hr; 191mph)
Max rate of climb at S/L, AUW as above: 378m (1,240ft)/min
Service ceiling, AUW as above: 5,610m (18,400ft)

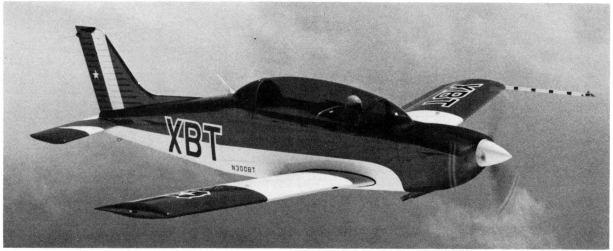
Piper PA-28R-300XBT Pillan.

Range with 45min reserves, AUW as above, 75% power, at 2,500m (8,200ft): 610nm (1,130km; 702 miles)
Range, econ cruising power, at 4,000m (13,100ft): 830nm (1,538km; 956 miles)

St Croix Ultralights Excelsior (USA)
Single-seat microlight
First flight: February 1982

The Excelsior is a very lightweight aircraft which qualifies for the FAA's non-licensed "ultralight" category or can be licensed under the "experimental" regulations applicable to homebuilt aircraft. Design and construction of the prototype began in September 1981 and the first flight was scheduled for February 1982. One of the Excelsior's main design features is its overwing-mounted engine, which drives a pusher propeller aft of the tail unit via a long drive shaft.

Powerplant: One 15kW (20hp) Zenoah Model 250
Wing span: 9.75m (32ft 0in)
Length overall: 5.03m (16ft 6in)
Weight empty: 82kg (180lb)
Max level speed: 78kt (145km/hr; 90mph)
Max cruising speed: 69kt (129km/hr; 80mph)
Econ cruising speed: 61kt (113km/hr; 70mph)
Max rate of climb at S/L: 213m (700ft)/min

Eipper-Formance Quicksilver Q-2 (USA)
Two-seat microlight
Introduced: February 1982

Suitable for training, photography and para-dropping, the Quicksilver Q-2 is a two-seat version of the earlier Quicksilver MX monoplane. It does not have the auxiliary fuel tank of the MX.

Powerplant: One 22.4kW (30hp) Cuyuna 430D
Wing span: 9.75m (32ft 0in)
Length overall: 5.51m (18ft 1in)
Weight empty: 127kg (280lb)
Max T-O weight: 318kg (700lb)
Max level speed: 39kt (72km/hr; 45mph)
Max cruising speed: 30.5kt (56km/hr; 35mph)
Econ cruising speed: 27kt (50km/hr; 31mph)
Max rate of climb at S/L: 107m (350ft)/min
Service ceiling: 3,050m (10,000ft)
Range with max fuel: 36nm (67km; 42 miles)
Endurance: 1hr 12min

Grob G-110 (West Germany)
Two-seat sporting aircraft
First flight: February 6, 1982

Grob-Werke began manufacturing sailplanes during the early 1970s. In 1982 it produced the G-110 two-seat powered monoplane, using glassfibre and other composites extensively in its construction. Series production was expected to begin in the summer of 1982.

Powerplant: One 88kW (118hp) Avco Lycoming O-235-M1 flat-four
Wing span: 10.60m (34ft 9¼in)
Length overall: 6.90m (22ft 7¾in)
Weight empty: 560kg (1,234lb)
Max payload: 240kg (529lb)
Max T-O weight: 900kg (1,984lb)
Max level speed: 151kt (280km/hr; 174mph)
Cruising speed (75% power) at 2,000m (6,560ft): 140kt (260km/hr; 162mph)
Max rate of climb at S/L: 288m (945ft)/min
Range with max fuel, 75% power: 647nm (1,200km; 745 miles)

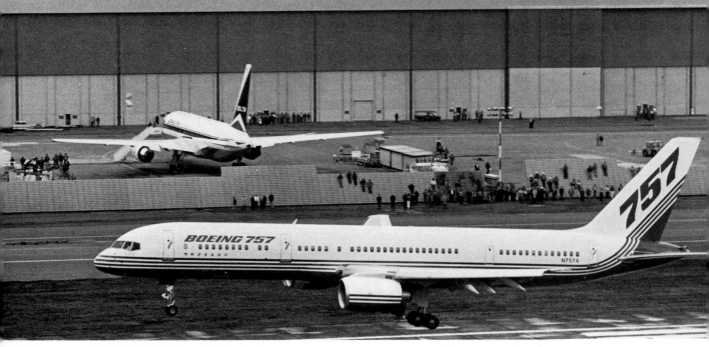

Boeing Model 757. *(Boeing)*

Boeing 757 (USA)
Short/medium-range airliner
First flight: February 19, 1982

In 1978 Boeing announced its intention of developing three new airliners, the Models 757, 767 and 777. The Model 757 is based on the Model 727 fuselage, improved performance coming from the use of two new high-bypass engines and an advanced-technology wing with less sweepback than that of the Model 727.

Eastern Air Lines and British Airways were the first to order the 757, contracting for 21 and 19 respectively in early 1979; both airlines also took out options on further aircraft. In March 1979 Boeing announced that full production had begun. The first 757 was rolled out at Renton on January 13, 1982, and flew the following month. Deliveries were scheduled to begin during December 1982. Those for Eastern Air Lines and British Airways are designated Model 757-200 and are to be powered initially by 166.4kN (37,400lb st) Rolls-Royce RB.211-535C turbofans. This is the first time that British jet engines had been used to launch a new Boeing airliner. The engines on Eastern aircraft are to be uprated later to –535E4 standard.

By March 1982 Boeing had received orders for 121 757s, with a further 56 on option, the largest number ordered being the 60 for Delta.

Powerplant: As above, or 170kN (38,200lb st) Pratt & Whitney PW2037, or 178.4kN (40,100lb st) Rolls-Royce RB.211-535E4 turbofans
Accommodation: Typical accommodation for 186 mixed-class passengers, or 204 in all-tourist configuration, or 239 maximum capacity
Wing span: 37.95m (124ft 6in)
Length overall: 47.32m (155ft 3in)

Weight empty (operating, with RB.211-535Cs and 186 passengers): 59,157kg (130,420lb)
Max T-O weight: 108,860kg (240,000lb)
Cruising speed (passengers and engines as above): Mach 0.80
Max range (passengers and engines as above): 2,070nm (3,836km; 2,383 miles)

Aérospatiale SA 365F Dauphin 2 (France)
Search and rescue and anti-ship helicopter
First flight: February 22, 1982

In October 1980 the government of Saudi Arabia ordered military equipment from France which included 24 SA 365F Dauphin 2 helicopters. Four were ordered as search and rescue helicopters with Omera ORB 32 radar, the remaining 20 as shore and frigate-based anti-ship aircraft equipped with Thomson-CSF Agrion 15 radar under the nose and Aérospatiale AS 15TT all-weather air-to-surface missiles (200 rounds ordered).

A full-scale mock-up of the anti-ship version was displayed in the same month that the Saudi order was placed, and the first SA 365F Dauphin 2 flew for the first time on February 22, 1982. Deliveries are scheduled to begin in 1983.

Powerplant: Two 530kW (710shp) Turboméca Arriel IC free-turbine turboshafts
Main-rotor diameter: 11.93m (39ft 1¾in)
Length of fuselage: 12.15m (39ft 10½in)
Max T-O weight: 3,900kg (8,598lb)
Radius of action (with two missiles): 165nm (305km; 190 miles)
Endurance: 2hr 45min and 3hr 45min with four and two missiles respectively

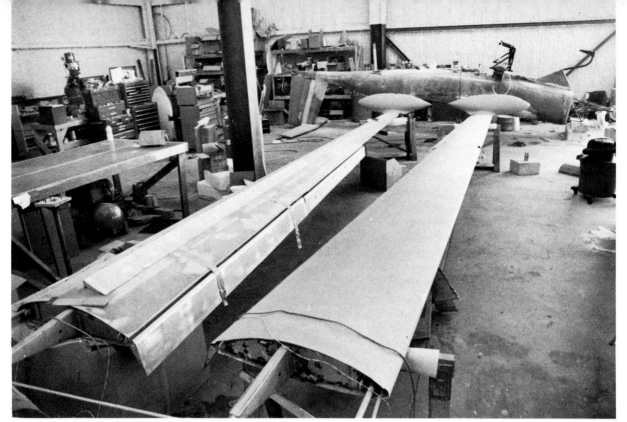

Free Enterprise **under construction, with fuselage in background and wings in foreground.** *(Howard Levy)*

Quickie Aircraft Corporation Free Enterprise (USA)
Single-seat record-attempt monoplane
First flight (in public): March 8, 1982

Originally known as *Big Bird*, *Free Enterprise* was designed and built by the Quickie Aircraft Corporation to attempt a non-stop flight around the world without flight refuelling. The future of the project was however thrown into doubt when Quickie Aircraft Corporation co-founder J. Thomas Jewett crashed and was killed while test-flying the aircraft on July 2, 1982.

Design of *Free Enterprise* began in 1978. It could carry 1,382lit (365 US gal) of fuel, which, because of the aircraft's outstanding efficiency, should have been enough for the record flight. If this had proved inadequate, however, the aircraft's modular structure would have permitted an increase to 2,082lit (550 US gal). The aerodynamics and powerplant could also have been changed. The entire flight was to have been made with power on. A full autopilot would have allowed the pilot to sleep for 10hr out of the estimated 90hr duration. A precise fuel totaliser would have performed fuel/drag/range calculations.

Powerplant: One 100.7kW (135hp) turbocharged Franklin/Pezetel O-235 flat-four
Wing span: 15.70m (51ft 6in)
Length overall: 7.52m (24ft 8in)
Weight empty: 771kg (1,700lb)
Max T-O weight: 1,928kg (4,250lb)
Cruising speed: 152-174kt (282-322km/hr; 175-200mph)
Estimated cruising altitude: 6,100-9,150m (20,000-30,000ft)
Max range: 21,276nm (39,430km; 24,500 miles)

Free Enterprise **in flight.** *(Hailey and Brown Advertising)*

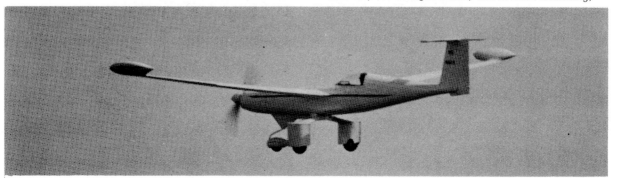

Airbus Industrie A310 (International)

Large-capacity wide-bodied short/medium-range transport

First flight: April 3, 1982

The A310 is a short-fuselage version of the successful A300, length being reduced by 13 frames. Cabin accommodation comes down to a maximum of 255 persons, although 210-234 will be normal. Fuselage cross-section remains unaltered, allowing two standard LD3 containers abreast and/or standard pallets installed crosswise. A new advanced-technology wing of reduced span and area is fitted, as well as new and smaller horizontal tail surfaces, new "multi-role" pylons able to support all the types of engine offered, and a modified landing gear.

At present the A310 is available in one basic version, the A310-200, for short/medium-haul operations, including transcontinental routes. However, further developments will eventually offer increased payload and range capabilities

Powerplant: Two 213.5kN (48,000lb st) General Electric CF6-80A1 (A310-202) or Pratt & Whitney JT9D-7R4D1 (A310-221), 222.4kN (50,000lb st) General Electric CF6-80A3 (A310-203) or Rolls-Royce RB.211-524B4 (A310-240), or 235.75kN (53,000lb st) Rolls-Royce RB.211-524D4 (A310-241) turbofans

Wing span: 43.90m (144ft 0¼in)

Length overall: 46.67m (153ft 1½in)

Typical operating weight empty: 76,616-76,895kg (168,910-169,525lb)

Max payload: 31,884kg (70,292lb)

Max payload (A310C-200 convertible version): 36,800kg (81,130lb)

Max payload (A310F-200 freighter version): 39,400kg (86,860lb)

Max T-O weight: 138,600kg (305,560lb)

Max operating speed: Mach 0.84

Typical high-speed cruise at 9,145m (30,000ft): 483kt (895km/hr; 556mph)

Typical long-range cruise at 11,275m (37,000ft): 447kt (828km/hr; 515mph)

Range with allowances, diversion and hold, max passenger payload (-202): 2,530nm (4,688km; 2,913 miles)

Range, conditions as above (-221): 2,470nm (4,577km; 2,844 miles)

Range, conditions as above, with max structural payload (-202, -221): 1,460nm (2,705km; 1,681 miles)

Range, conditions as above, with max fuel (-202): 3,510nm (6,504km; 4,041 miles)

Range, conditions as above, with max fuel (-221): 3,490nm (6,467km; 4,018 miles)

Airbus Industrie A310. *(MBB)*

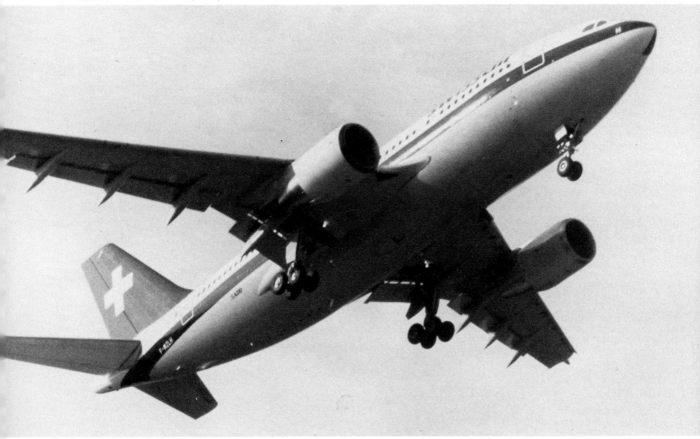

Canadair CL-601 Challenger (Canada)
Business, cargo and commuter transport
First flight: April 10, 1982

The CL-601 is the newest version of the Challenger, fitted with two 38.48kN (8,650lb st) General Electric CF34-1A turbofans. It made its first flight in April 1982, and production deliveries were expected to start in the second quarter of 1983. By March 3, 1982, a total of 142 Challengers had been ordered, and 40 CL-600s completed.

Powerplant: See above
Accommodation: Up to 19 passengers
Wing span: 18.85m (61ft 10in)
Length overall: 20.85m (68ft 5in)
Weight empty: 9,054kg (19,960lb)
Max T-O weight: 18,892kg (41,650lb)
Max cruising speed: 488kt (904km/hr; 567mph)
Time to 13,715m (45,000ft): 22min
Max certificated operating altitude: 13,715m (45,000ft)
Range with reserves, standard fuel: 3,700nm (6,857km; 4,260 miles)

Sikorsky S-76 Military (USA)
Military helicopter
First flight: April 1982

This is a military development of the S-76 Utility. It incorporates the latter helicopter's armoured crew seats, heavy-duty floor and sliding cabin doors but is also equipped with a weapons pylon, an optical sight mounted above the instrument panel, self-sealing high-strength fuel tanks, and provision for weapons fired from the doors.

In May 1982 the prototype conversion completed weapon-firing demonstrations with 7.62mm Minigun and M-60D machine guns fired from the doors, SU-11A and TMP 7.62mm gun pods, and 2.75in folding-fin rockets carried on the pylon.

The following details refer to the S-76 Mark II, the current (from March 1982) production version of the civil helicopter.

Powerplant: Two 508.5kW (682shp) Allison 250-C30S turboshafts
Main rotor diameter: 13.41m (44ft 0in)
Length of fuselage: 13.22m (43ft 4½in)
Weight empty, standard equipment: 2,540kg (5,600lb)
Max T-O weight: 4,672kg (10,300lb)
Max cruising speed at 4,536kg (10,000lb) AUW: 145kt (269km/hr; 167mph)
Max rate of climb at S/L: 411m (1,350ft)/min
Service ceiling, weight as above: 4,570m (15,000ft)
Range with 12 passengers, standard fuel, 30min reserves: 404nm (748km; 465 miles)

BAe VC10 K2 (UK)
Military flight-refuelling tanker
First flight: June 22, 1982

In 1978 the British Government decided to investigate the feasibility of converting ex-civil VC10s into flight-refuelling tankers for the RAF. After a design study

BAe VC10 K2. *(BAe)*

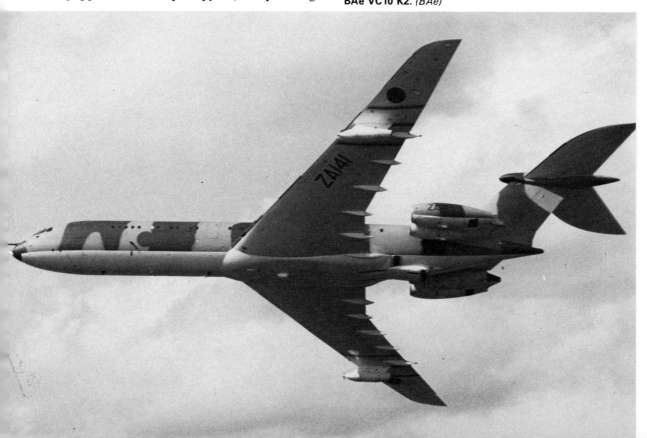

nine aircraft were acquired for this conversion. Five of the nine were standard Model 1101s built for BOAC, and the other four were the Model 1154 Super VC10s delivered to East African Airways. After conversion these will be known as K2s and K3s respectively. To supplement the nine K2/3s when the RAF's Victor tankers have been retired the 13 VC10 multi-mission transports currently serving as VC10 C1s with No 10 Sqn are to be modified for a secondary tanker role.

Powerplant: Four 97kN (21,800lb st) Rolls-Royce Conway Mk 550B turbofans, interchangeable with the Conway 301s installed in the VC10 C1
Accommodation: Flight crew of four. Limited rear-facing seating provided for airlift of essential ground personnel when the tanker is deployed away from its home base; K2 seats 18 persons, K3 17. Forward underfloor freight hold is unchanged and can be used to carry spares or refuelling pods during ferry flights. Fuel for flight-refuelling operations is accommodated in five cylindrical tanks installed within the fuselage. These tanks and the aircraft's basic fuel system are interconnected, and it is possible to transfer all but the fuel needed for the tanker's mission, and to take on fuel through a nose-mounted probe
Wing span: 44.55m (146ft 2in)
Length overall (K2): 48.36m (158ft 8in) excl refuelling probe

Laker: The Man Who Fell to Earth

ALAN W. HALL and SUE BUSHELL

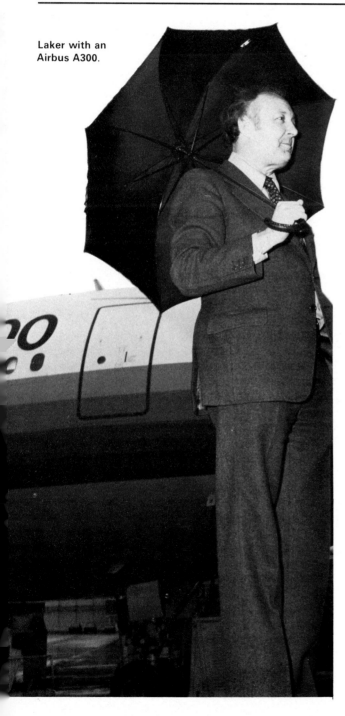

Laker with an Airbus A300.

On a cold winter's morning in January 1965 a group of about 50 aviation and travel journalists assembled at Gatwick Airport at the request of a man whose star was at that time very much in the ascendancy in airline circles. Freddie Laker was becoming well known for his co-operation with the press, and he could always be relied on for a good story and a few juicy quotes. As head of British United Airways, Laker intended to show exactly what he wanted to do with the latest British-built airliner, the BAC One-Eleven. At that time no other airline had shown any interest in buying the type, and it was left to the Americans and British United to show how good the aircraft was. The One-Eleven could have had no finer advocate than Freddie Laker.

By the time the first light of dawn had crept over the Gatwick horizon the journalists were airborne in One-Eleven G-ASJI, bound for Genoa. In under two hours they were being well looked after at the best hotel in town, before being flown back to London. A short while later they were on their way again, this time to Paris, where after a 35min turnround the One-Eleven headed back to London. "This," said Freddie Laker, "is the way I am going to use this aircraft." After six hours' flying the journalists were equally convinced that British United could fly their new aircraft to the limits, changing crews and keeping the aircraft longer in the air than on the ground.

Throughout the journey to Genoa and then Paris, Freddie Laker was constantly on his feet, talking to his guests, explaining about the virtues of the aircraft and making sure they had their fair share of the liquid refreshment provided. He did a first-rate public relations job which set the One-Eleven and British United well on the way to getting as much scheduled and charter business as they could handle over the next decade.

Freddie Laker's background is a varied one. After RAF service during the war he became associated with Aviation Traders at its Southend base. It was there that Laker made his first big purchase when in 1948 the company acquired BOAC's entire fleet of Handley Page Haltons, converting them for use by the smaller charter companies engaged in the Berlin Airlift. Bond Air Services of Southend became the largest user, with

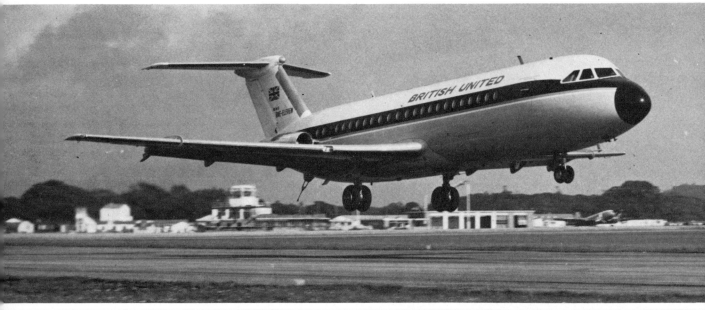

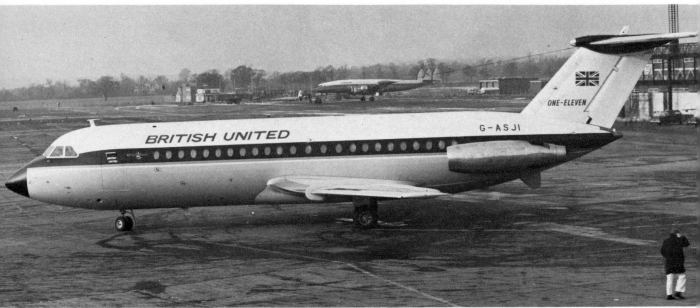

Top **The prototype BAC One-Eleven, painted in British United livery from its very first flight.** *(Vickers-Armstrong)*

Above **One-Eleven G-ASJI, used to carry the press on a whirlwind tour in January 1965.** *(BAC)*

---

12 aircraft. By the time Bond withdrew from this work it had completed no fewer than 2,577 sorties and flown almost 6,500 hours. In 1949 Capt Bob Treen and Freddie Laker founded Skegness (Airport) Ltd, and Bond operated charter flights on behalf of the airport. Business fell off, however, and by 1951 Bond had ceased trading.

The Prentice market cornered
But Laker was still interested in buying aircraft and converting them for civilian use. His next venture was

with the Percival P.40 Prentice, which became surplus to RAF requirements in 1955. Aviation Traders bought almost the entire stock of obsolete machines, flying them into Southend and Stansted to await conversion. No fewer than 252 were delivered, of which only 28 eventually found civil employment. Laker's aim was to produce a "people's aeroplane" which would be cheap to buy and would revolutionise British general aviation. Unfortunately, the cost of conversion, the high operating charges and the restrictions placed on Aviation Traders by the authorities meant that the venture was not a success.

Thanks to its continuing maintenance work, Aviation Traders remained in business in spite of the losses that must have resulted from the Prentice affair. Then came another new idea: why not build a new aircraft from scratch? Aviation Traders duly designed and built the ATL.90 Accountant, a 28-seat airliner powered by two Rolls-Royce Dart 512 turboprops. Registered G-ATEL, the prototype was first flown on July 9, 1957, and appeared at the Farnborough Show in September of the same year. Aviation Traders promoted the design as yet another replacement for the DC-3/Dakota, but the number of seats was wrong for the market and the economics of the new airliner did not meet expectations. Development work was eventually abandoned in January 1958.

By 1959 work had started on the ATL.98 Carvair, intended as a follow-on from the Bristol Freighter, which at that time was making a lot of money for Channel Air Bridge and Silver City Airways as a quick, cheap and efficient way of taking cars to Europe. Surplus DC-4s were bought and Aviation Traders rebuilt the forward fuselages, allowing room for five average-sized cars and 25 passengers at a fraction of the cost of a new aircraft.

Below **Aviation Traders Accountant G-ATEL**. *(APN)*

Bottom **Under Laker's guidance British United adopted the VC10 with an enlarged freight door on the port side**. *(BAC)*

Looking beyond the Carvair

Work on the first Carvair (G-ANYB) began at Southend in 1960, by which time Laker was looking ahead once more. March of that year saw proposals for the merger of Hunting-Clan and Airwork, along with a number of associated companies. The merger came into effect on July 1, 1960, and the new group was named British United Airways. Channel Air Bridge and Silver City were also involved in the merger, and it was therefore natural that Laker would play a significant part. He became managing director of the new company, which soon showed signs of being the largest of the British independent airlines. New routes and aircraft were acquired, business in the form of trooping contracts and charter work flowed in, and the company prospered under the day-to-day guidance of the dynamic Laker. Then came the establishment of Air Holdings, formed to control the interests of British United. Laker was appointed a member of the board: he had finally achieved the public and corporate recognition he sought.

BUA was the first carrier to order the BAC One-Eleven for internal, European and medium-haul scheduled services. The airline also bought VC10s for

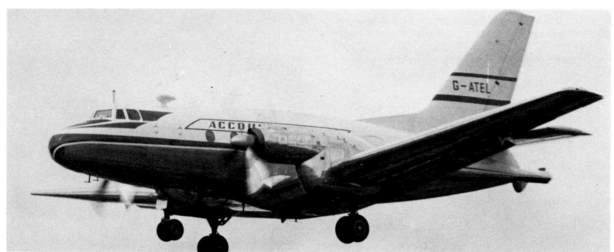

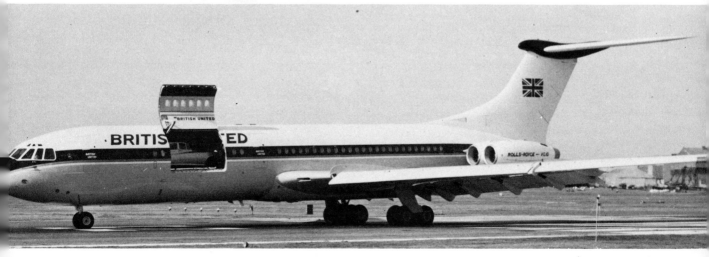

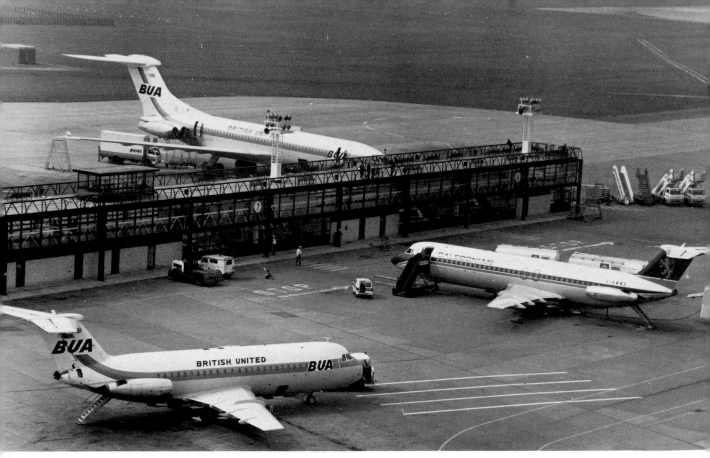

Predating the merger of BUA and Caledonian, this photograph shows a BUA One-Eleven and VC10 in company with a Caledonian One-Eleven. *(BAC)*

long-haul routes, and competed with the major flag carriers in every way.

But Laker wanted his own airline so that he would be free to put to the test his ideas about making air travel cheap and easily accessible to everybody. Laker Airways was eventually formed in February 1966 as a contract hire and ad hoc charter organisation based at Gatwick and operating two former BOAC Britannias. Three BAC One-Eleven Series 300s were immediately ordered, though when the first was delivered it was sold at once to Lord Brothers for that company's inclusive-tour programme, on which it flew close to 1,700hr during its first year of operation. The second One-Eleven was leased to Air Congo for a period, and the Britannias found work with a number of airlines, including Air France.

Laker tail: DC-10-10 G-AZZC
Eastern Belle.

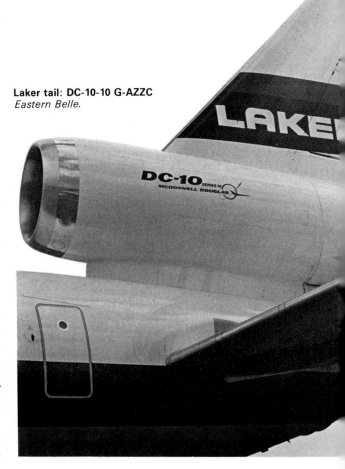

Laker on the up and up

Laker then acquired Arrowsmith Holidays, sold the Britannias, bought Boeing 707s and started operations from Berlin for German holidaymakers. The 707s were ideal for transatlantic charters, and Laker entered this market in 1969. At the end of that financial year Laker was able to announce a record pre-tax profit of £482,687 and a passenger total of 335,272, 40 per cent up on the first year of operations.

By 1970 Laker Airways had become a large organisation and there was speculation that British United

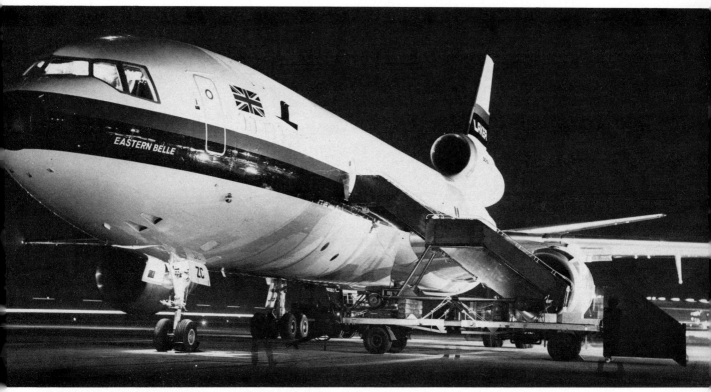

Used for ad hoc charters throughout Europe before the trans-atlantic services began, G-AZZC is seen at RAF Wildenrath, West Germany, on December 18, 1972, after completing a Christmas trooping flight. *(RAF)*

would be acquired when it came up for sale that year. Caledonian Airways eventually bought United, however, and Laker had to content himself with setting up International Caribbean Airways in September 1970 and starting a scheduled 707 service between Luxembourg and Barbados.

The first ultra-cheap transatlantic flights came in 1971, when Laker applied to the Department of Trade and Industry for a licence to fly a no-reservation "Skytrain" 707 service between Gatwick and New York. The original single fare was to have been no more than £37.50 at the height of the summer season. The application for traffic rights was denied but, with the setting up of the Civil Aviation Authority in April 1972, he tried again, suggesting that Douglas DC-10s would be used. This time the licence was granted, with the stipulation that Stansted be used instead of Gatwick as the UK terminal. Two new Douglas DC-10-10s were ordered, the first arriving in November 1972. Proving flights were made to every UK airport offering enough runway length to permit safe operations.

Laker was intent on pursuing his policy of offering the sort of prices that would make air travel even more popular, bringing low fares into areas hitherto governed by Iata airlines, which in his opinion fixed prices unnecessarily high. But the necessary permission from the American authorities was slow to come, and before Skytrain started the two DC-10s were used on charter flights to various European destinations. Then the government of the day withdrew official approval of the routes and fares, leaving Laker with three idle DC-10s — a third aircraft had meanwhile been delivered — on his hands. For two and a half years these aircraft, although under-utilised, were employed on charter work throughout Europe and to the United States.

Skytrain takes off
The breakthrough eventually came and the British public and their American opposite numbers responded enthusiastically to the offer of cheap, no-frills transatlantic travel, much to the disgust of some of the longer established airlines on the route. Few people will forget the long queues at London's Victoria Station, at Gatwick and New York when the first services were operated. Some travellers had to wait several days before they eventually got on board, but that did not matter all that much because the low fare and the feeling of history in the making more than made up for any inconvenience. Freddie Laker became, almost overnight, a public figure and people welcomed his defiance of entrenched authority and championing of free enterprise.

However, the writing was on the wall even then, for the financing of Laker by major world banks relied on the strength of sterling against the dollar. Nevertheless, Laker went ahead and inaugurated new routes: there was no holding him now. Los Angeles was the next gateway to fall, though routes to Canada were not as profitable.

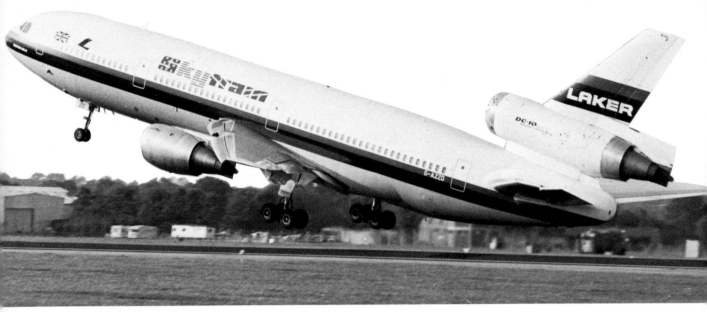

Laker's Skytrain motif was painted on the fuselage of this DC-10-10 before licences had been granted for the Atlantic service. *(APN)*

Laker at the Toulouse Airbus A300 production line.

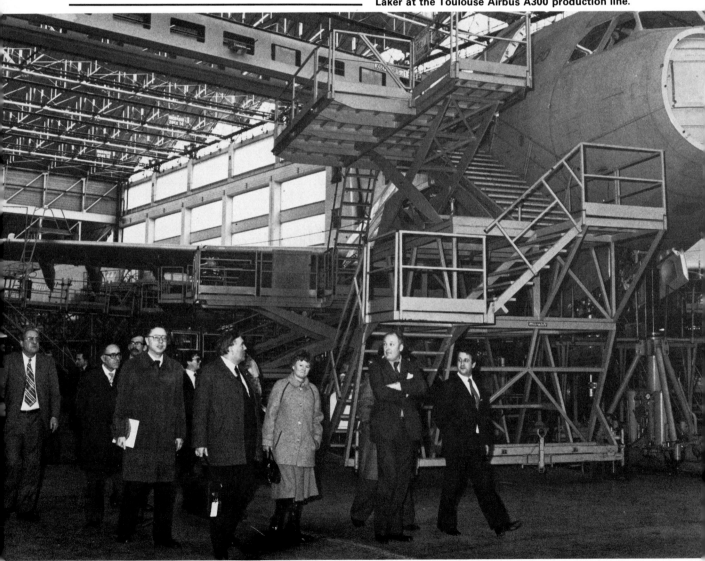

Laker also saw his chance to provide Skytrain-style services on popular European routes. He applied for and eventually achieved a scheduled service to Zurich. Other routes were also in the offing and, working in the belief that he would get his way in the end, Laker looked at the Airbus A300 as his next aircraft type.

He went to Toulouse, placed orders and forecast at a press conference that he was the man who would really make the A300 pay. After all, the manufacturer's name neatly summed up his philosophy of making air travel cheap enough for everybody to enjoy. Ten A300s were ordered for delivery between 1981 and 1984, and with them Laker intended to open up the charter market and cut his European fares way below those of the nearest competition.

Not surprisingly, the airlines which were forced to lower their fares in the face of Laker competition were not slow in responding to the threat. No one can say that they ganged up against Laker, but by offering cut rates on Atlantic services they were able to compete even though they knew that, by their standards, they were operating at a loss. Laker set up an advance booking system so that his passengers did not have to wait in a queue before they got their seats. But the other airlines were only marginally more expensive by this

The first Laker Airways Airbus A300, still carrying a French registration. *(GIFAS)*

time and to some extent traffic fell away, particularly during the winter months.

The cracks begin to show
At this point rumours that all was not well within the Laker camp began circulating. By autumn 1981 it was known that because of the increase in value of the dollar the repayments on loan capital were behind and that Laker was asking for more time. Loans in the region of £130 million were at stake, and although spokesmen for the company affirmed that the payments on six of the DC-10s in the fleet had by that time been almost completed, this was not the whole story. There were also the remaining five still to be paid for, plus $31 million outstanding on the A300 fleet.

Such figures are not uncommon in the world of airline financing, so why was Laker forced into liquidation? Perhaps the simple answer is that Laker, who had been knighted by that time, remained insistent that his company should be independent. He almost scorned a bail-out with public money, and in the event a last-minute change of heart met with official indifference, such was the Thatcher Government's insistence on its "no lame ducks" policy.

Negotiations were put in hand during December 1981 to get a year's deferment of the loan repayments. In the meantime, Sir Freddie stated that he was fore-

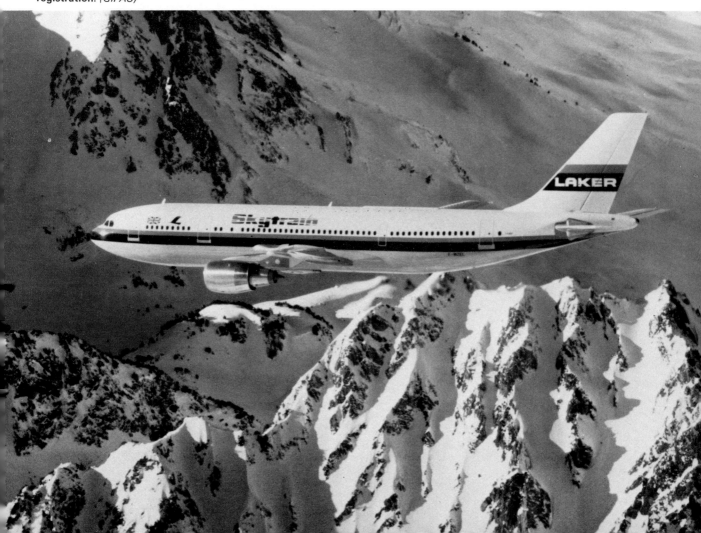

casting a £15 million profit for the year, though it was not made clear whether this was operating or net profit. Then came a major restructuring of Laker's finances which resulted in Sir Freddie's losing much of his 90 per cent shareholding, and companies like McDonnell Douglas and other creditors becoming shareholders. For a time this seemed likely to save the business, for it was seen as of little use to reclaim the aircraft and sell them elsewhere, such was the depressed state of the airliner market.

The furore died down over Christmas, but in January 1982 it became known that the European finance houses had said that Laker must sell off his A300s and that at least 10 per cent of the existing staff must be made redundant. There was the possibility that the A300s then in service would be kept on until the end of the 1982 summer season, as this operation would be profitable and would help to pay off the mounting debts. Fares too would have to be increased if the bankers were to be satisfied.

It seemed that Laker, whose confident air on television helped inspire a public will to back him, was still in difficulties, and that a restructuring of the Atlantic routes mooted for later in the year would be greatly to the disadvantage of the airline.

The crash comes

The crash came on February 5, when operations ceased abruptly just after 10 a.m. The airline announced that it had been forced to call in the receiver and that its aircraft were immediately grounded. One aircraft with a party of prospective holidaymakers aboard was in fact recalled in mid-flight.

Within hours of the liquidation announcement, the British public's regard for Sir Freddie Laker became evident as a fighting fund was established in an attempt to save the company. By the end of the day £1,000,000 had been donated, including gifts from passengers who had been turned away at check-in desks and had their holidays ruined.

Laker's collapse was discussed in Parliament the same afternoon, when it was revealed that a last-minute appeal had been made to the government for financial aid and that this had been rejected. Labour members also called for an urgent review of British aviation policy.

But was Laker finished? After a few days in seclusion he was back again trying to raise his company from the ashes. When it became clear that this was impossible he put forward a new scheme: a "people's airline". With negotiations going on between himself, the Lonrho company and city bankers, there was just a chance that this might come to fruition despite strong opposition. It was not to be, however, and the profitable parts of the Laker empire, including the travel organisations, were sold off, leaving the world's airlines to breathe a sigh of relief that the thorn in their side had departed. Ironically, Laker's aircraft have now been sold to companies such as British Caledonian, which had opposed him in so many licensing battles. His routes across the Atlantic have also been redistributed, again in some cases to British Caledonian, and the once-proud Laker placard has gone from the maintenance area at Gatwick.

Have we seen the last of Sir Freddie Laker? Possibly not. Public memory is short and soon many will probably not even remember the crisis that arose within the British airline industry during the 1981-82 winter. Though Sir Freddie Laker may have retired from public life for the time being he could yet return with one more scheme for making air travel available to the widest possible market.

A Light Touch on the Controls

DAVID MONDEY

The years between the end of the Second World War and 1982 have seen spectacular improvements in the capability of both civil and military aircraft. This results from a combination of factors that include advances in aerodynamics, structures, materials and engines. The first flight to exceed a speed of Mach 1 was recorded by Capt Charles Yeager USAF in the Bell X-1 (initially XS-1) rocket-powered research aircraft on October 14, 1947. Just over six months later this speed was attained in a dive by the turbojet-powered North American YF-86A Sabre prototype. Within six years the North American F-100 Super Sabre, the first turbojet-powered fighter capable of Mach 1 in level flight, was entering service.

For a number of years there was no let-up in the quest for ever more speed in air-superiority fighters, but combat experience in South-east Asia was to bring a better appreciation of the need for highly efficient all-weather radar, effective missile armament, and higher manoeuvrability, whether at the expense of speed or not. The last-named trade-off posed many problems, leading initially to compromise and later to new thinking on the subject of flight control. In America airborne computers and inertial measuring units had been developed for the control system of the Apollo Lunar Modules that carried men to and from the Moon's surface during 1969-72. It seemed that an application of this system could offer a great deal to the control of conventional aircraft operating in the Earth's atmosphere, ensuring fast and accurate positioning of the aircraft's control surfaces. More important, it was believed that the computer/sensor combination would be able to set control surfaces at the optimum position more effectively than a human pilot. This could lead to a reduction in the basic weight and drag of aircraft, offering increased payload and flight performance. To appreciate how this might be achieved, it is necessary to look at the way in which flight controls have developed.

The problem of control
Even before sustained powered flight became a reality in 1903, there had been many people concerned with the problem of finding an effective control system for the new machine when it eventually became airborne.

Indeed, there already existed a significant body of experience of flight, much of it gained by the German pioneer Otto Lilienthal. Between 1891 and his death on August 10, 1896, Lilienthal made more than 2,000 flights, all accomplished with his beautifully constructed lightweight gliders. They had no controls and were true hang-gliders, with the pilot supported by his arms so that he was free to move his body and legs in any direction. By this means he could shift the aircraft's centre of gravity (CG) to achieve some degree of control in pitch, roll and yaw. The degree of control was of course very limited, but Lilienthal was learning by experiment and practice the nature of the problems involved. Understandably, he worked towards making his aircraft inherently stable, so that flight could be accomplished with a minimum of body movement. However, by late 1895 he was already formulating ideas for the more practical forms of flight control that his own experience had shown would be needed, especially when powered flight became a reality. But in this respect even Lilienthal's pioneering work had been antedated: the British pioneer Sir George Cayley had used fixed tail controls, a rudder and elevator, to achieve a successful flight by his model glider of 1804.

Even more interesting, perhaps, is the fact that at the time of Lilienthal's achievements, and even earlier, men such as France's Charles Renard and the American Hiram Maxim were thinking seriously about automatic flight control. Renard is known best in aviation history for his association with Arthur Krebs in the development of the electrically powered airship *La France*, first flown in 1884. He had experimented in 1873 with an unmanned multi-wing glider that incorporated a transverse pendulum mechanism which, if the aircraft began to roll, would actuate small control surfaces, one on each side of the aircraft, to bring it back to an even keel. Maxim evolved a far more advanced mechanism incorporating a gyroscope suspended as a pendulum to provide control in pitch, and he intended to use and assess this "stabiliser" in conjunction with the enormous biplane test rig which he built in Baldwyn's Park at Bexley, Kent. When tested for the third time on July 31, 1894, the biplane was damaged and he terminated his experiments. As a

113

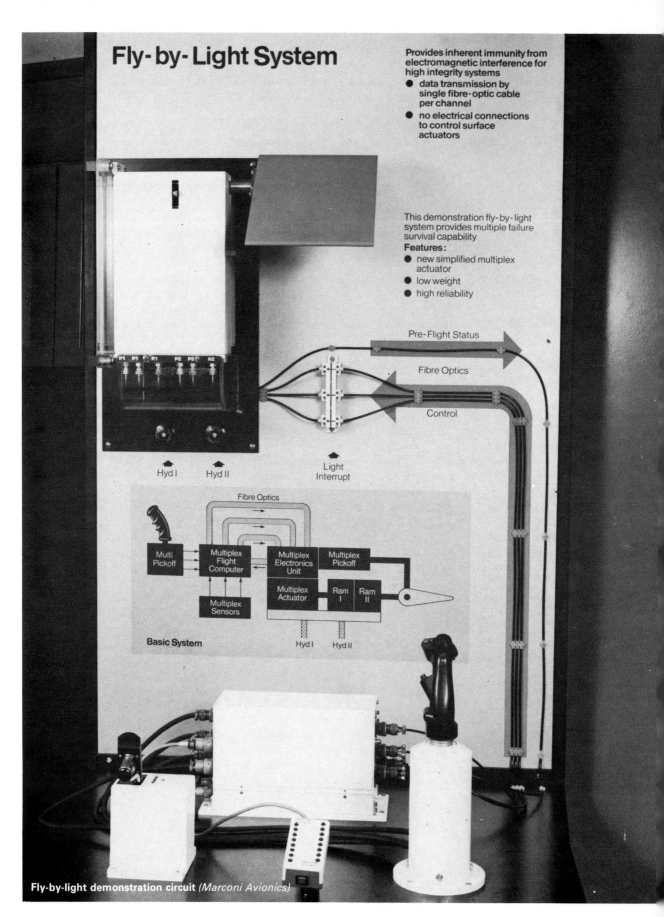

Fly-by-Light System

Provides inherent immunity from electromagnetic interference for high integrity systems
- data transmission by single fibre-optic cable per channel
- no electrical connections to control surface actuators

This demonstration fly-by-light system provides multiple failure survival capability

Features:
- new simplified multiplex actuator
- low weight
- high reliability

Pre-Flight Status

Fibre Optics

Control

Hyd I   Hyd II   Light Interrupt

Fibre Optics

Multi Pickoff

Multiplex Flight Computer

Multiplex Electronics Unit

Multiplex Pickoff

Multiplex Sensors

Multiplex Actuator

Ram I   Ram II

Hyd I   Hyd II

Basic System

Fly-by-light demonstration circuit *(Marconi Avionics)*

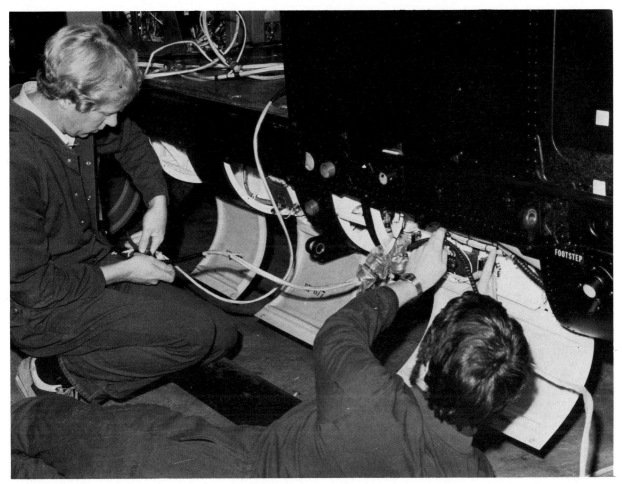

Trial installations of fibre-optic looms on a Westland Lynx helicopter. *(Westland)*

result, the very advanced stabiliser was abandoned without practical test.

With most pioneers working towards a very stable aircraft that would stay on a more or less even keel once airborne, that Wright brothers adopted a totally different approach. They sought an aircraft that would border upon being unstable, requiring the provision of efficient controls to make it stable and to give the pilot authority over the flightpath, allowing him to choose his course through the air. Powered flight duly became a reality, and control of the aircraft in pitch and yaw relied in general upon surfaces called elevators and rudders respectively. Control in roll was achieved by the Wright brothers through wing warping, but ailerons, small hinged surfaces incorporated into the wing structure, were soon shown to be far more effective. These three traditional forms of control surface have stayed the course to date, albeit with improvements and the addition of new surfaces and devices to augment them.

Putting the pilot into the loop
How does the pilot move these surfaces to control the aircraft in flight? Initially, flexible wire cables linked the pilot's stick and rudder bar with ailerons/elevators and rudder respectively. The control cables were light in weight and fairly easy to route throughout the airframe; unfortunately they stretched and frayed and needed a lot of maintenance. More practical, but heavier and more complicated, were push-pull rods. Many systems of both types survive to this day, often in combination. Effective control links became even more important as aircraft grew in size and control-surface loadings increased. Gradually a variety of trim systems were introduced to reduce the aerodynamic loads on control surfaces that made it difficult or tiring for the pilot to hold the aircraft in straight and level flight. These loads can vary greatly on commuter services, for instance, as the number of passengers changes from stage to stage, or on military aircraft as fuel is consumed and weapons expended. Both civil and military operations result in CG shifts that change the aerodynamic loads on control surfaces. This problem gave rise to the development of automatic flight control systems capable of maintaining the aircraft in level flight and on a set heading.

Higher speeds, higher wing loadings and demands for greater manoeuvrability all added their quota to the complexity of control systems. And when aerodynamic trim systems could no longer cope with the loads,

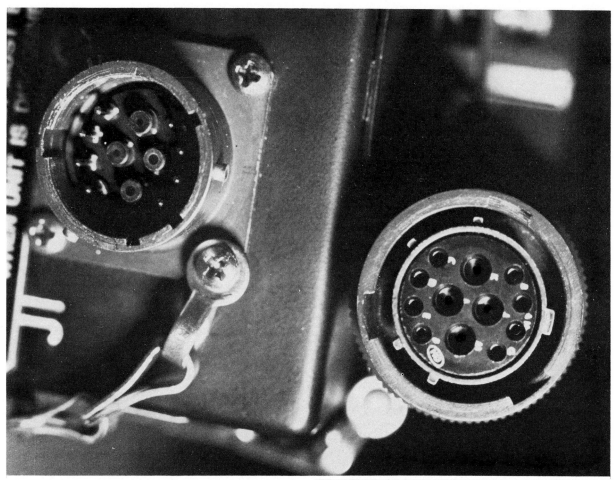

Marconi-developed fibre-optic connector. *(Marconi Avionics)* | **Advanced fibre-optic connectors.** *(Marconi Avionics)*

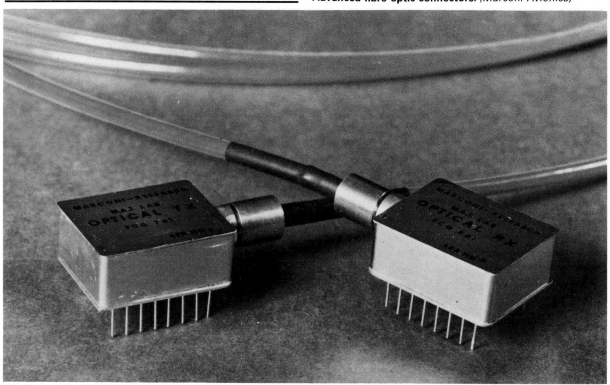

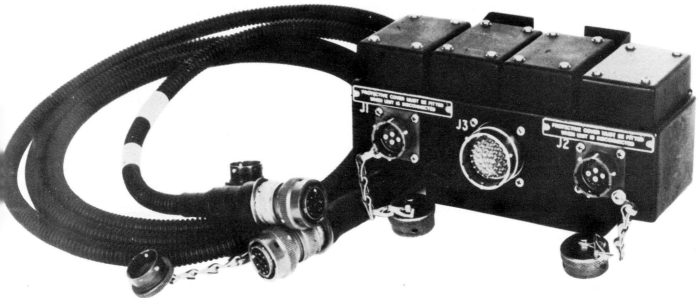

Optical coupler unit for the Boeing YC-14 transport. *(Elliott Brothers)*

power-assisted controls were introduced. In a typical example of such a system hydraulic actuators operated the actual surfaces, with the pilot's controls routed via and interconnected with hydraulic boosters. This ensured that if the booster system failed, the pilot could still retain manual control over the aircraft. As control loadings became still higher, fully powered systems were introduced, with the pilot's control column given artificial "feel" so that he still received a physical impression of the effects of moving his controls.

The complexities of supersonics

The development from the mid-1950s of supersonic military aircraft made entirely new demands of aircraft controls, requiring faster response and back-up systems. In fact, the steady development of multiple-redundant flight control systems stems from this period. Multiple redundancy is a "belt and braces" approach to flight control: in the event of failure or destruction of a control link there is an alternative to fall back upon. Simple redundancy was often incorporated in early aircraft controls by the duplication of flexible wire cables — the hope was that both would not be severed simultaneously — and in power-assisted systems there was simple reversion to manual control in the event of hydraulic system or booster failure.

Clearly, however, there are limits to the amount of redundancy that can be built into an aircraft. The rapid approach of these limits, and the quest for more manoeuvrability, led to extensive research into systems which would link electronically the pilot's controls and the aircraft's control surfaces. At the heart of such systems lies a computer able to integrate the inputs received from the pilot's controls and equipment sensing the dynamic forces acting upon the aircraft, and almost instantly signal the control surfaces to the optimum position. From this work have resulted safe and practical fly-by-wire (FBW) systems that create a relationship between pilot and aircraft response which is always acceptable to both man and structure.

FBW duplicates the flexible cables that once linked pilot and control surfaces, and in some recent applications replaces them completely. There are of course aircraft with FBW systems in which limited manual reversion is retained: this is usually applied to the elevators, ailerons or pitch and roll-control spoilers, to give the ability to return to base or make a successful forced landing. These variations apart, an FBW system comprises wires carrying electric signals that link the pilot's controls, via microcomputers, with the electro-mechanical actuators that move the control surfaces.

Marconi Avionics Ltd of Rochester, Kent, can look back on more than two decades of highly successful work in the field of advanced flight control. The company's work has resulted in high-integrity automatic flight control systems for a variety of aircraft, including the Anglo-French Concorde and the British BAe One-Eleven, VC10, Buccaneer, Harrier, Lightning, Lynx and TSR.2. But the first genuine FBW to enter production was the company's system for the Tornado. This has "pure" FBW control of rudder and spoilers, with mechanical reversion for taileron control in the unlikely event of a complete electronics failure. Marconi also developed the full FBW system for the Boeing YC-14 Stol transport prototypes. The current pinnacle of FBW development is the integrated flight control system (IFCS) for the UK Jaguar FBW demonstrator programme. A major design requirement was that this highly advanced system should be at least as reliable (expressed as the probability of total system loss) as the mechanical control linkages that it would replace.

Handling qualities to order

Why is FBW better than the advanced autopilots that it supersedes? Whereas an autopilot provides only flightpath guidance, enabling the pilot to fly hands-off while he carries out other tasks, FBW defines the very relationship between movement of the pilot's controls and the aircraft's response. The system is never disengaged, and it determines the aircraft's handling qualities throughout each flight. One significance of airborne computers is the fact that they can make the handling qualities acceptable over a wide flight envelope. Another is that, provided with a means of defining the aircraft's handling qualities via the controls, the designer has a new freedom to choose a shape which is aerodynamically most efficient. In seeking greater fuel economy, higher speeds or larger payloads, the designer has hitherto been compelled to produce an aerodynamic shape which leads to good handling. Such shapes can mean a high structure weight and, at the same time, cause high drag. With FBW the structure can be designed so that performance aims take priority, leaving the flight control system to take care of the handling qualities. The pilot has to make no change in the way in which he handles the controls, but the resulting aircraft is far more efficient.

The ultimate in flight control?

Does this mean that FBW represents the ultimate in flight control systems? The answer is no, for FBW can be vulnerable to lightning strikes or the gamma rays generated by tactical nuclear weapons. The resulting loss of control might only last a fraction of a second, but could be fatal for aircraft operating at high speed close to the ground or in close formation. Protection from such short-term electromagnetic surges can be achieved by shielding or "hardening" the system, but this could add greatly to weight and cost.

Marconi Avionics has developed a practical alternative to FBW which is immune to electromagnetic surges. In the company's fly-by-light (FBL) system conventional wire circuitry is replaced by optical fibres through which data are transmitted in the form of light. Early Marconi FBL systems embodied optical fibres composed of multiple filaments, but the recent development of single-filament fibres means that, compared with FBW, FBL now offers significant weight savings and greater system efficiency. Details of the signal generators and receiver/actuators are a commercial secret, but it is clear that Marconi's FBL handles data far more quickly than any other system. Furthermore, there are no electrical connections between the signal transmitter and the control surface actuators. Even more interesting is the fact that, by using light of different wavelengths and adopting filter-separation techniques, it is possible to transmit simultaneously several streams of data through a single filament.

Fly-by-light earns its wings

Marconi's advances in the field of FBL have not been limited to research and development. In late 1972 Boeing and McDonnell Douglas each received US Air Force contracts for the construction of two Advanced Medium Stol Transport (AMST) prototypes for competitive evaluation. Boeing's two YC-14 AMSTs made their first flights within ten weeks of each other, in August and October 1976. They incorporated an Electrical Flight Control System (EFCS) that was fundamentally FBW. The heart of that system was the Flight Control Electronics (FCE) system developed by Marconi Avionics (then known as Marconi-Elliott Avionics Systems Ltd) and incorporating fibre-optics to transfer data between three computers via interface units for the purpose of inter-lane voting. The system proved to be thoroughly practical and reliable, and more than met the requirement.

Research and development is a continuing process, but Marconi Avionics already has a practical FBL system available when needed. The advantages of the use of FBL for the designer of military aircraft — weight savings, immunity to electromagnetic pulse, resistance to battle damage, high manoeuvrability — are manifold. But its application to the world's fleet of passenger transports may prove far more important, resulting in greater efficiency, reliability and flight safety.

This is the Age of the . . . Biplane?

KENNETH MUNSON

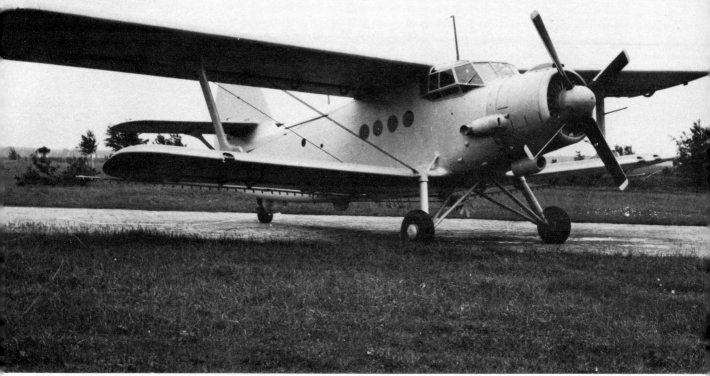

Antonov An-2 in agricultural form.

Pick up any general account of the aviation scene written in the middle to late 1930s and the chances are that it will, directly or by implication, include somewhere the sentiment that "the days of the biplane are numbered". At that time there seemed little reason to doubt such a view, for it was the age of sleek new 300mph (483km/hr) monoplane fighters like the Spitfire, long-range giants such as the Flying Fortress, and of airlines queuing up to buy the new range of fast, modern airliners from Douglas, Boeing and Lockheed.

The ensuing six years of war did little to dispel the notion that the biplane was a design of the past, despite the often heroic exploits of such obsolescent stalwarts as the Gladiator and Swordfish. It may therefore come as a surprise that the current editions of *Jane's All the World's Aircraft* contain descriptions of more than 50 different types of biplane, many of them of quite recent design. None of course is a candidate for commercial transport or military duties, but the biplane, instead of

becoming obsolete, has simply moved further into areas where its particular attributes still make it a good choice.

Most of the biplanes produced today are within the realm of homebuilt and sporting aviation, but nearly a dozen types form a part — often a leading part — of one of the busiest, most important and most rapidly expanding areas of general flying: agricultural aviation. Doyen of them all is the An-2, still in production 35 years after its first flight in 1947. Output to date has included more than 5,000 by the Antonov factories in the Soviet Union, where it was designed, followed by more than 9,000 at WSK Mielec in Poland, which took over the production line from the USSR in 1960. Probably another thousand or two have been built in the People's Republic of China, where it also remains in production. The An-2 performs a truly wide variety of different duties, though well over half of the 15,000 or more built have been put into service as cropsprayers and dusters.

119

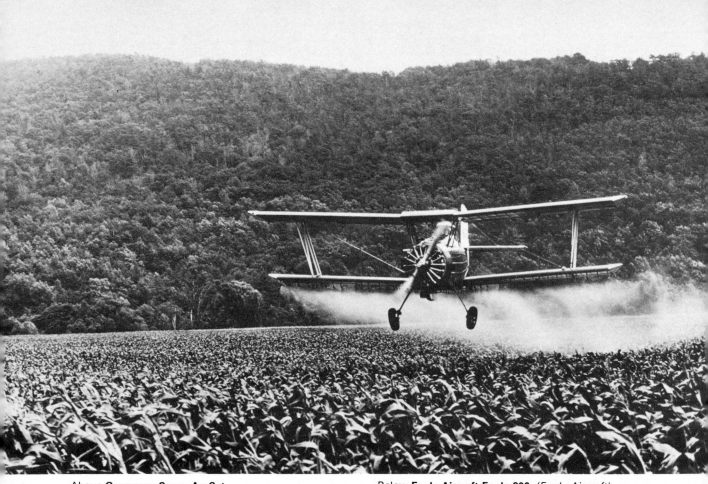

Above **Grumman Super Ag-Cat.**　　　　　　Below **Eagle Aircraft Eagle 300.** *(Eagle Aircraft)*

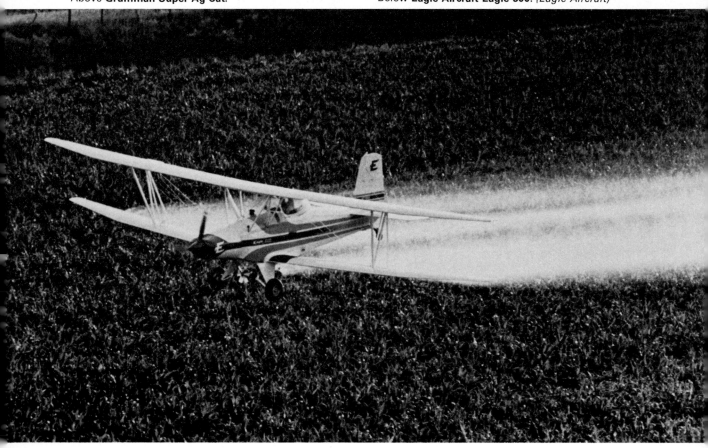

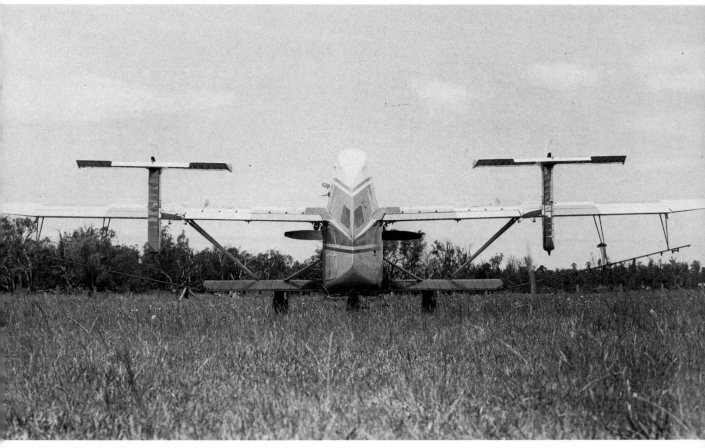

Rear view of the Transavia Airtruk T-320. *(Transavia)*

The hazards of agricultural flying

Agricultural flying is a highly specialised and inherently hazardous occupation, demanding extremely low-level flying, tight turns and maximum controllability at very low speeds. More often than not it has to be carried out in the tricky half-light of early morning or evening, when the pests to be destroyed are least active. It calls for a special breed of pilot, and for the safest and most controllable aircraft available. A manufacturer's description of the Ag-Cat, another of the most widely used "aggies," gives an idea of some of the advantages which make the biplane so suitable for this exacting role: "Low take-off and landing speeds materially reduce the possibility and severity of accidents . . ., the two sets of wings and attaching structure will absorb more than twice the crash energy of a monoplane's single set of wings and structure . . .abrupt stalls simply do not occur . . .gentle stall, combined with superb manoeuvrability and light control forces, makes the least possible demands on pilot skill, and is less likely to induce pilot fatigue . . .excellent speed-control characteristics inherent in the biplane's design keep re-entry speed within reasonable, safe limits . . .uncanny ability to turn in a small, tight radius after a run and get back down over the field is a function of its biplane configuration . . .the correct wing arrangement of a biplane gives it the stability needed to make an extremely tight turn with complete safety."

Grumman designed the Ag-Cat in the mid-1950s, subcontracting its manufacture in 1957 to Schweizer Aircraft Corporation, which was still building the current B-Plus versions in 1982, having turned out nearly 2,500 "aggies" in 23 years. In addition, conversions known as the Turbo Cat and King Cat are being produced by Marsh Aviation and Mid-Continent Aircraft Corporation respectively, the former with a 447kW (600shp) turboprop and the latter with an 894kW (1,200hp) radial replacing the 335.5 or 447kW (450 or 600hp) radial of the standard versions.

The An-2 and Ag-Cat are both thoroughly conventional, but some other crop-control biplanes show varying degrees of design ingenuity. In Argentina Aero Boero found it worthwhile to turn its successful little AB 180 cabin monoplane into a biplane, as the 180 SP, utilising the lower pair of wings as integral tanks for 330lit (72.5 Imp gal) of liquid chemical, which in the previous AB 180 Ag version was stored in a bulky underfuselage pod. In America in the late 1970s the Eagle Aircraft Company of Idaho designed a brand-new biplane, also called the Eagle, which has long-span (16.76m; 55ft) narrow-chord wings with upper-surface spoilers that owe much to modern sailplane technology and have integral spraybooms forming the trailing edge

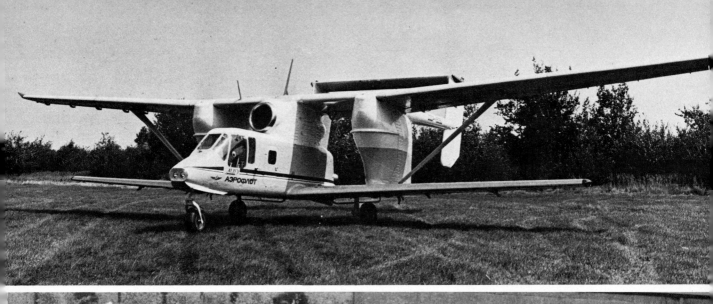

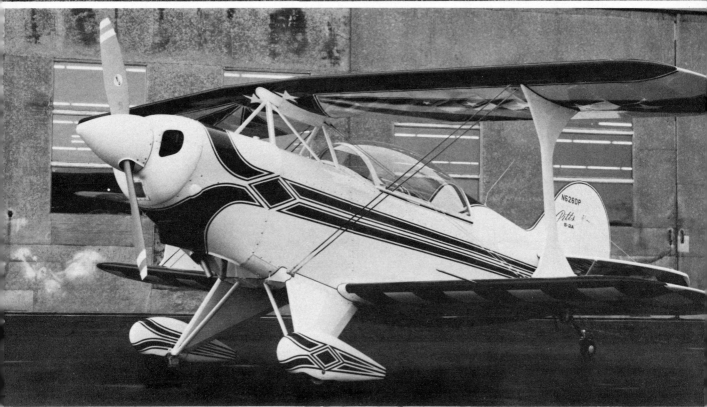

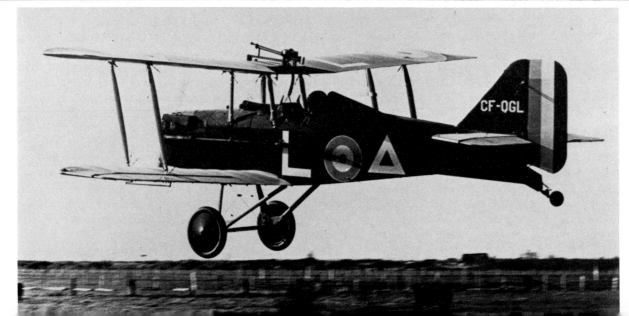

of the lower wings. Another thoroughly unorthodox type is Transavia's Airtruk, an Australian design of the mid-1960s. Strictly a sesquiplane, or "one-and-a-half-wing" biplane, the Airtruk has a unique configuration. Twin (but unconnected) tailbooms and tail surfaces allow a road vehicle to drive up and load chemical directly into the hopper in the pod-shaped central nacelle.

The unique, unorthodox Belphegor

Also unique, and perhaps the most unorthodox of all modern biplanes, is Poland's M-15 Belphegor, produced by the WSK (Transport Equipment Manufacturing Centre) at Mielec. Together with the An-2 and two monoplane designs, the Kruk and Dromader, the Belphegor was one of four types of agricultural aircraft produced in Poland (production has recently ended). Intended as the mainstream successor to the An-2, it was designed jointly with the USSR, which indicated a requirement for as many as 3,000 examples. When Soviet designer R. A. Ismailov and his Polish colleague

K. Gocyla assembled their two-nation team at Mielec to develop the M-15, they decided at a very early stage that a large biplane would provide the best answer to their requirements. They then reasoned that, since they would have to brace the two sets of wings anyway, why not do so with a structure that could at the same time accommodate the substantial load of chemical which the aircraft had to carry? The result was a pair of long, deep and narrow hoppers located quite close to the fuselage sides and occupying the entire gap between the upper and lower wings. The two hoppers can carry a combined load of 2,900lit (638 Imp gal) of liquid or 2,200kg (4,850lb) of dry chemical fed directly into a dispersal system which forms an integral part of the lower wing trailing edges. A single strut outboard of each hopper is the only other support needed to brace the Belphegor's 22.33m (73ft 3in) span upper wings. The aircraft is also unique in one other respect: it is the only agricultural aircraft in the world, and the only biplane, to be powered by a turbofan engine. It received a full Soviet certificate of acceptance in April 1979.

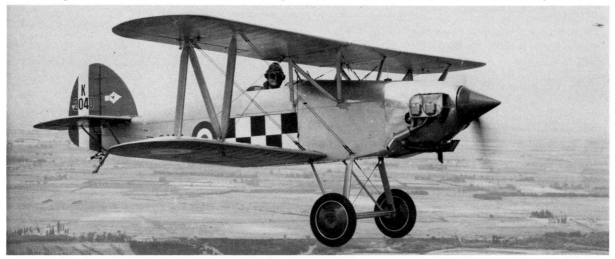

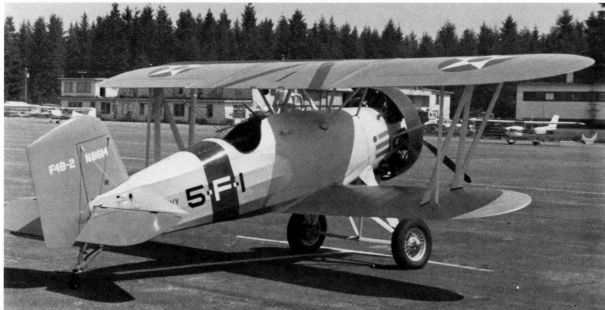

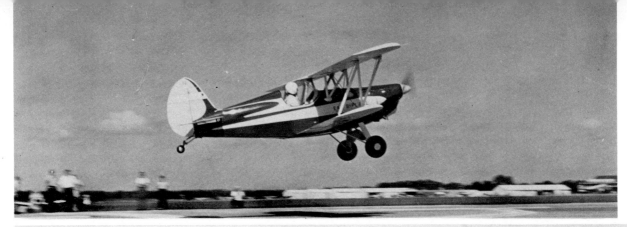

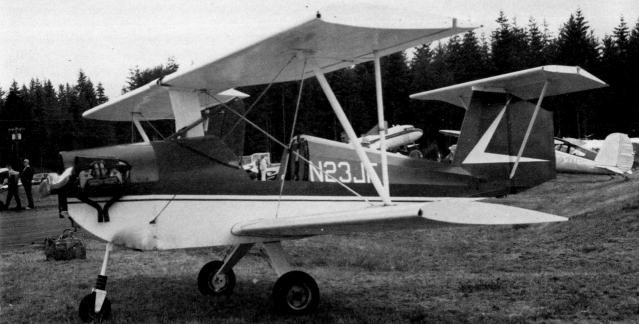

Top **EAA Biplane.**

Above **Aerosport Scamp A.** *(Peter M. Bowers)*

Apart from farm pilots, others keen to enjoy the delights of "wind in the wires" flying can find more than 40 different types of biplane from which to choose in the current pages of *Jane's All the World's Aircraft.* Anyone who has seen the Pitts Special thrown about the sky in aerobatic competitions, or watched the polished performances of the Rothmans aerobatic team, will need little further convincing of this tiny aeroplane's truly outstanding controllability and performance. A real old-timer, of which nearly 150 latter-day examples have been produced, is the Great Lakes Sport Trainer. First built in 1929 with a Cirrus or Menasco engine, it reappeared in the early 1970s with an Avco Lycoming engine (currently of 134kW; 180hp) and such modern improvements as a constant-speed propeller, inverted fuel and oil systems, and ailerons on both upper and lower wings. Approved aerobatic manoeuvres include spins, chandelles, lazy eights, loops, barrel rolls, primary rolls, point rolls, slow rolls, snap rolls, Cuban eights, hammerhead and Immelmann turns, and split Ss — surely enough to satisfy the most demanding of pilots.

Homebuilt hot ships

But the happiest hunting ground of all for the would-be biplane flyer lies within the prolific field of homebuilt designs, which range from "golden oldies" to quite modern designs. If his taste is for a near-replica of a genuine fighter of bygone days, he can choose plans and/or construction kits for a First World War S.E.5A from Replica Plans in Canada, a Hawker Fury from John Isaacs in the UK, or a Boeing F4B from Aero-Tech in the USA. A 1914-18 flavour with a dash of originality can be found in Donald Stewart's Foo Fighter, with its distinct overtones of the Bristol F.2B, or Marshall White's Der Jäger, which has major assemblies patterned on the wings of the Albatros D.Va, main landing gear fairings of the Focke-Wulf Stösser, and tail unit of the Fokker D.VII.

Those preferring to build a more conventional and well established pair of wings may opt for plans of the EAA Biplane (over 7,400 sets sold) or Acro-Sport (nearly 1,000 sets), Peter Bowers' Fly Baby (which began as a monoplane in 1960 and became available optionally as a biplane eight years later), or one of the many variations of Vernon Payne's delightful 1928-designed Knight Twister. Barney Oldfield will be

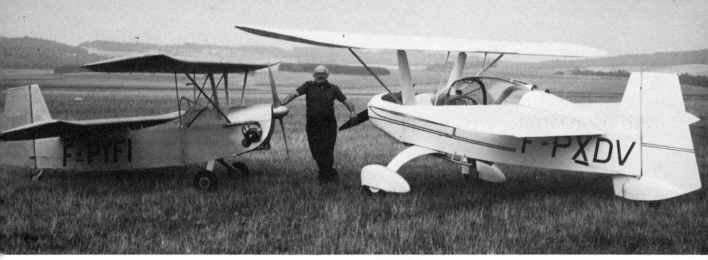

Above **Landray GL01 two-seater (right) and smaller GL02.**

Below **Thompson Boxmoth.**
(Thompson International)

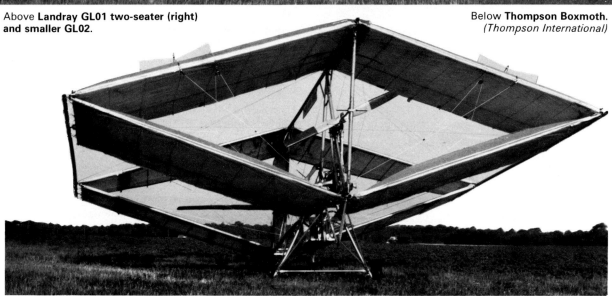

Smith DSA-1 Miniplane.

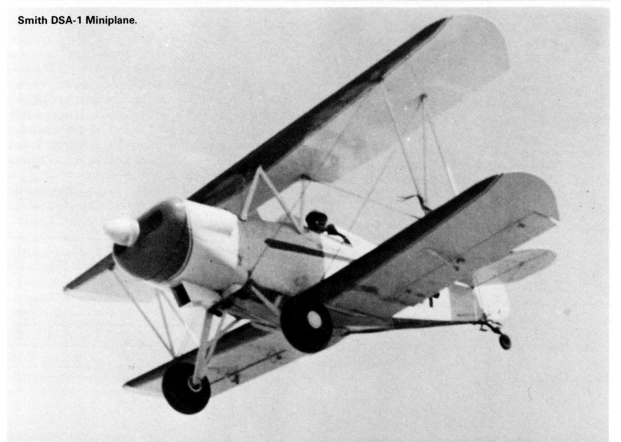

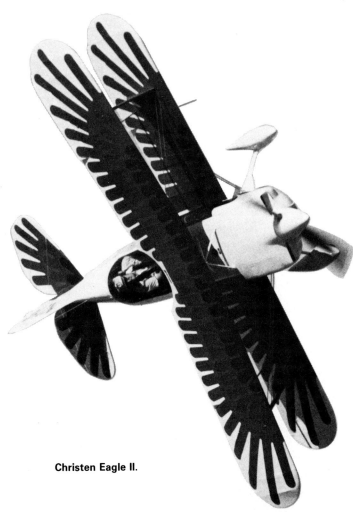

Christen Eagle II.

An even more strange-looking tandem-wing design is the Boxmoth ultralight developed by Richard R. Thompson of Philadelphia, which has wings of rhomboid planform. Strictly patented by Mr Thompson, and available for construction only under his specific licence, the Boxmoth can be built without any welding, machining, sheet metal, woodwork, conventional fabric or dope, using materials readily available from local hardware, farm supplies and recreational vehicle dealers. Any high-performance, lightweight snowmobile, motorcycle or outboard engine can be fitted, the prototype having a 41kW (55hp) snowmobile powerplant. Wings and tail are covered with Mothsilk nylon-reinforced vinyl, the wings being foldable so that the aircraft can be towed on a car trailer and stored easily. Gross weight for take-off is only 238kg (525lb).

Small is desirable

Smallness is also a deliberate ingredient of the Smith Miniplane (its DSA-1 designation stands for Darn Small Aeroplane), a 454kg (1,000lb) single-seater capable of 217km/hr (135mph) on an 80.5kW (108hp) engine; it can accommodate other powerplants rated at up to 93kW (125hp). A dozen or more other US homebuilt biplanes include the fully aerobatic Christen Eagle; Nicholas D'Apuzzo's Freshman and Senior Aero Sport; William Durand's unstallable Durand Mk V with negative-stagger wings; the Volkswagen-engined Der Kricket from Flight Level Six-Zero in Colorado Springs; the neat, two-seat Hatz CB-1, two/three-seat Javelin Wichawk and two-seat Laven LACO-125; the two-seat aerobatic Hiperbipe (HIgh PERformance BIPlanE) from Sorrell Aviation, and Skybolt from Steen Aero Lab; and Stanley Wallis's unusual Red Wing Black Bird.

The newly fledged crop of microlight aircraft also includes a number of biplane designs. UFM's Easy Riser and its solar-powered Solar Riser variant, Michael Fisher's Flyer and Barnstormer, Jim Jaeger's J-Bird, and Bob Hovey's Whing Ding II and slightly larger Delta Bird head the US designs, while MEA in England has recently created the Micro Bipe for British enthusiasts and others. And those who want a biplane but don't require an engine at all can join the 200 or so other amateurs in the Bahamas, Brazil, Japan and the USA who are building ex-USAF Colonel William L. Skliar's Explorer Aqua Glider.

Sport and agricultural flying are among the most intensively performed aviation activities in the world, but the biplane's attractions do not end there. The Massachusetts Institute of Technology, which has a long and enviable record of contributions to aeronautical advancement, chose a biplane configuration for its

pleased, on the other hand, to sell plans of one of his three "Baby" versions of the Great Lakes Sport Trainer. Aerosport, in North Carolina, offers the comparative rarity of a tricycle-gear biplane with its Scamp A (also built, incidentally, in Colombia for agricultural work as the Scamp B). And the 1957-designed Stolp Starduster two-seater is still going strong, as are its more recent aerobatic stablemates, the single-seat Acroduster and two-seat Acroduster Too.

In Europe popular designs include the BA-4B and BA-11 from veteran Swedish designer Björn Andreasson, the latter having a choice of open or enclosed cockpits, and the lightweight (408kg; 900lb gross weight) Currie Wot, with a 48.5kW (65hp) Walter Mikron engine, for which plans can be obtained from Britain's Popular Flying Association. The influence of Henri Mignet lives on in France in the form of no fewer than seven current tandem-wing types (biplanes lifted by two wings in tandem, neither bearing more than 80 per cent of the total weight): the Pouplume and Criquet of Emilien Croses, Gilbert Landray's GL01, 02 and 03, the Lederlin 380-L, and Claude Piel's twin-engined push/pull C.P.500. They range in size from under 272kg (600lb) for the Pouplume to a 1,500kg (3,307lb) take-off weight for the yet to be completed five-seat, enclosed-cabin C.P.500.

Top **Hatz CB-1**.

Middle **LACO-125**.

Right **UFM powered Easy Riser**. *(Howard Levy)*

126

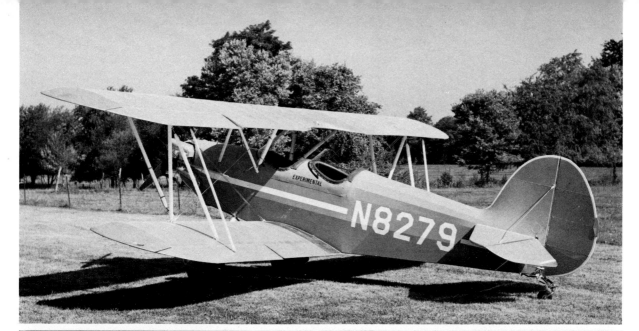

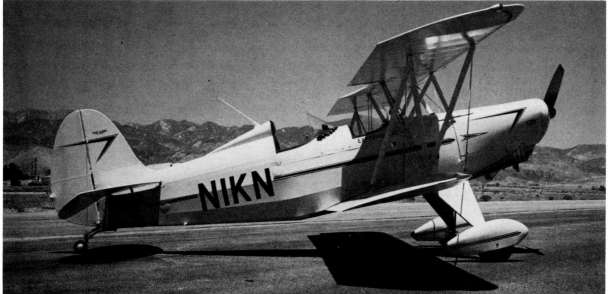

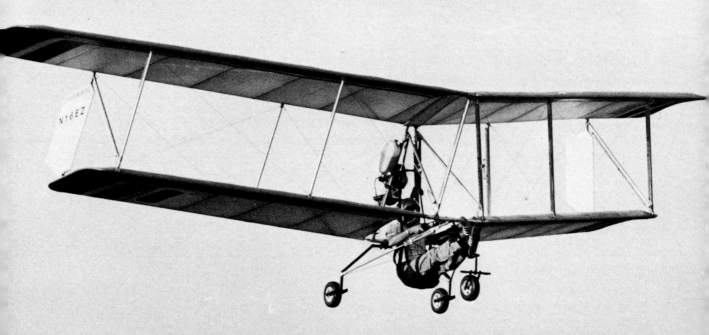

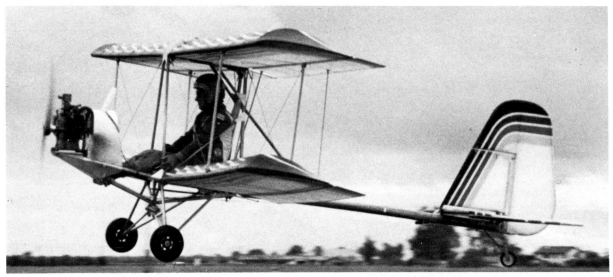

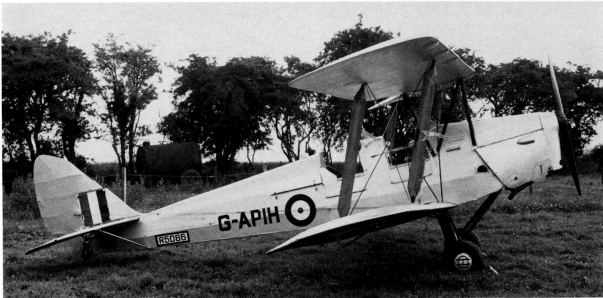

Top **Hovey Delta Bird**. *(Howard Levy)*

Above **Tiger Moth**. *(Peter J. Bish)*

1978-79 man-powered aircraft programme. Known as the Chrysalis, this made 345 flights, including several turns, in the hands of 44 pilots during its brief life.

Many other biplanes, although no longer in current production, can be found on the civil registers of practically every country. They vary from world-famous types like de Havilland's Tiger Moth to carefully nurtured veterans such as the sole surviving Grumman FF-1. Finally, there is one very special biplane which, although it has long ceased to exist, still has its name included year after year in each new edition of *Jane's*. This is the Caproni Ca 161*bis*, a modest little Italian "bipe" which, on October 22, 1938, powered by a 522kW (700hp) Piaggio radial, carried pilot Mario Pezzi to a world height record of 17,083m (56,046ft). In 44 years no other piston-engined aircraft, monoplane or biplane, has been able to improve upon that achievement.

Fly Met

MICHAEL J. H. TAYLOR

It was in 1921 that London's Metropolitan Police first went airborne, when officers observed the crowds and traffic on Derby Day from the R33 dirigible. In 1934 trials were conducted with an autogyro, and from 1967 with helicopters, leading to the extensive use of chartered helicopters from 1973.

In 1979 alone the helicopter unit of the Metropolitan Police answered 1,623 emergency calls, flying 1,217hr and achieving in the arrest of 246 people. Such successes had to lead to greater things, and in 1980 the Met became the first police force in Britain to buy a helicopter for surveillance work. In the first nine months of operation the newly acquired Bell 222 flew 1,061hr and participated in the arrest of 350 persons.

This aircraft and the second Bell 222 that has followed it into service are no ordinary helicopters. Hailed as the world's most sophisticated police helicopter, the first cost £600,000, plus £150,000 to equip it for traffic and crowd surveillance, escort and protection, emergency situation co-ordination and the many other roles it can be called on to perform. The most spectacularly evident of these systems are Heletele (see page 59), mounted in a pod on the starboard stub wing, and a Decca TANS F12 computer-display navigation system, while an infra-red camera is available for the detection of buried bodies or criminals in hiding. Also capable of accommodating eight persons or stretchers, the Bell 222s of the Met's Air Support Unit certainly lengthen the long arm of the law.

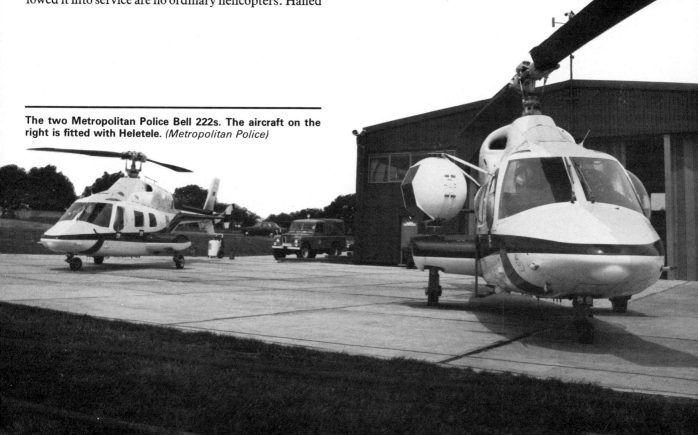

The two Metropolitan Police Bell 222s. The aircraft on the right is fitted with Heletele. *(Metropolitan Police)*

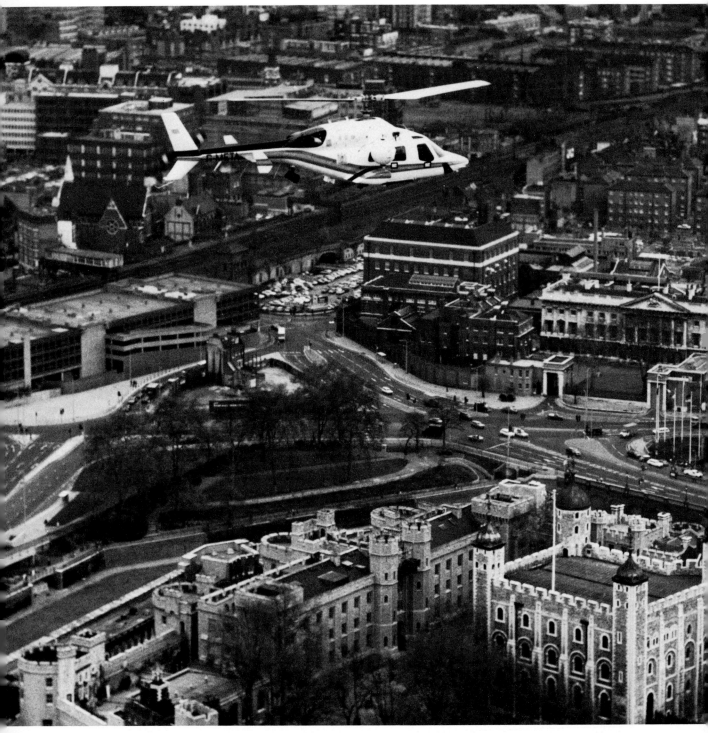

The first Met Police Bell 222 flying over central London. *(Metropolitan Police)*

Top right **A change of role necessitates a change of equipment: this Bell 222 carries a loud-hailer system and Nightsun floodlight.** *(Metropolitan Police)*

Right **Flight deck of a Met Police Bell 222.** *(Metropolitan Police)*

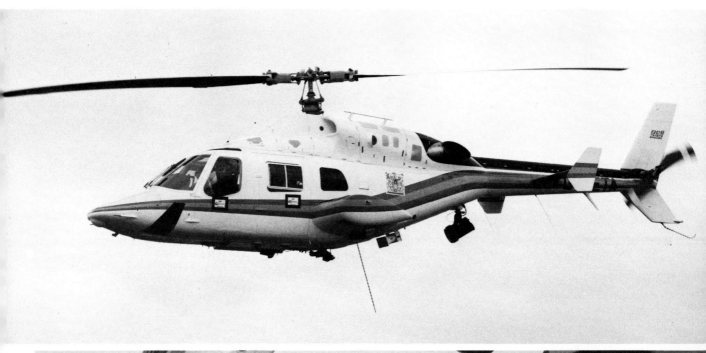

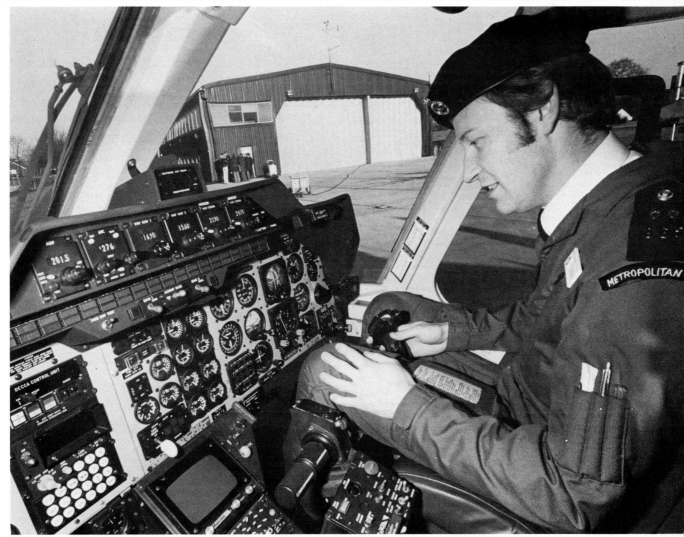

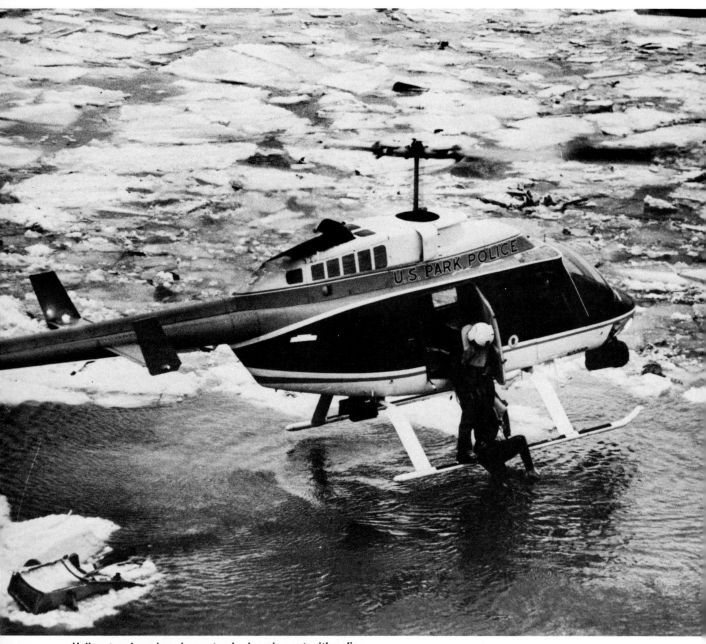

Helicopters have long been standard equipment with police forces in the United States. Here a Bell LongRanger II helps in the recent rescue of survivors from an airliner crash in Washington's Potomac River.

Methane: Aviation's Answer to the Oil Squeeze?

PHILIP JARRETT

Prompted by escalating Avgas costs, the Beech Aircraft Corporation of Wichita, Kansas, is evaluating liquefied methane gas as a potential substitute fuel for aircraft. A modified Beech Sundowner powered by an Avco Lycoming O-360 engine rated at 134kW (180hp) when using Avgas has been tested to determine the feasibility of using methane as an aircraft fuel. The key parameters studied were: the horsepower available when using liquefied methane, the cooling characteristics in various climb conditions, and the modified aircraft's range and endurance.

Methane offers several advantages over Avgas. It costs about half as much and, being a part of natural gas, is in abundant supply. It can also be obtained from coal gas and sewage. US Coast Guard investigations suggest that in comparison with other fossil fuels, methane is safer, clean-burning, and harmless to health and the environment. Its ignition temperature is much higher than that of Avgas, and it burns only within a narrow range of fuel/air ratios. Moreover, it is claimed that oil contamination and carbon build-up in piston engines is virtually eliminated, greatly extending the time between major overhauls.

In 26 years of providing cryogenic systems for Nasa manned space missions, Beech amassed a great deal of expertise in dealing with liquefied gases. The company began experimenting with the adoption of methane for cars in the early 1970s. Experience gained from the automobile system, now marketed by Beech, provided the basis for the equipment fitted in the Sundowner. Three additional engine components are needed: a modified carburettor, a pressure regulator, and a heat exchanger. The system is centred on a Beech cryogenic storage tank (like those in which hydrogen and oxygen were stored in Nasa's Apollo, Skylab and Space Shuttle programmes), which works like a super vacuum flask to keep the methane at −260°F. Between the inner stainless steel tank holding the fuel and the carbon steel outer tank is a super-insulation material. The tank is so efficient, say Beech engineers, that it would keep a cup of coffee hot for ten years. Since all air in the tank is displaced by liquefied methane and its vapours, the fuel is non-combustible and there is less danger in the event of a tank rupture.

The Sundowner's fuel tanks were positioned behind the front seats, the fuel being vaporised by the heat exchanger and raised to near-ambient temperatures. At the fuel/air mixer, which replaces the usual carburettor, fuel is reduced from its storage pressure of 1.38-2.07 bars (20-30lb/in²) to a pressure of 0.138 bars (2lb/in²).

Following initial tests with Avgas to provide comparative data, the methane system was ground-tested, the engine's timing having been adjusted to reduce

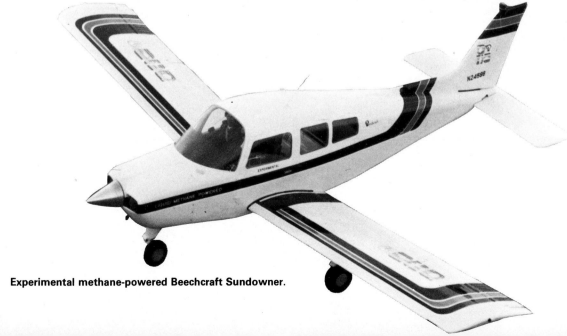

Experimental methane-powered Beechcraft Sundowner.

133

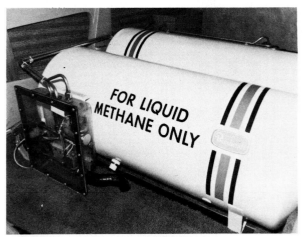

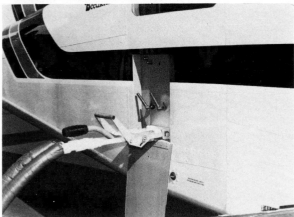

exhaust gas temperatures. These trials suggested that there would be a 10 per cent power reduction but that specific fuel consumption would be some 15 per cent less. The modified aircraft first flew on September 15, 1981, and made its public debut at the company's 1982 annual sales conference.

Although it is unlikely that an adequate liquefied methane distribution system could be in operation before the turn of the century, Beech believes that flying schools, corporate shuttles and commuter airlines could be the first to benefit from the use of the new fuel. It is reasoned that a large flying school could gain an early advantage by having its own fuel installation to serve its fleet of aircraft.

As if to back its claims, Beech has converted many of the cars and trucks in its Wichita fleet to liquid-methane operation. Naturally, the process of research, testing and eventual certification will take time, but the company firmly believes that the looming energy problems will be greatly eased by the perfection of aviation methane.

Top **Twin 18gal liquid methane tanks replace the rear seats in the experimental Sundowner.**

Left **Liquid methane is pumped into the Sundowner through this quick-connect fuelling coupler. The fuel enters via the input line in a liquid state and is vented as a gas through the return line when the tanks are full.**

Below **Instrument panel of the experimental Sundowner. The two large dials at lower right are used to monitor temperatures and pressures at various points in the fuel system.**

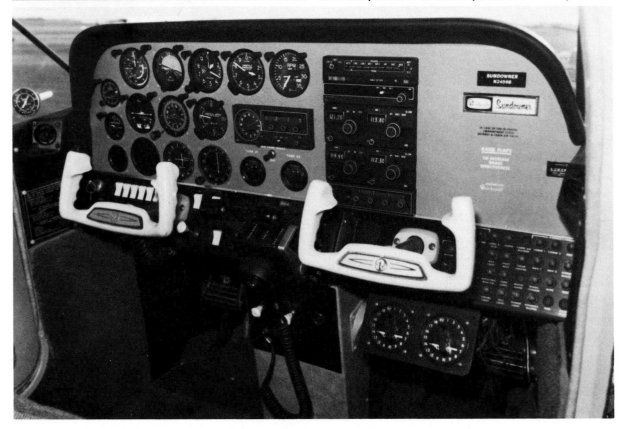

Flying Boats for the 1990s

ROY McLEAVY

An aerodynamic phenomenon which enabled scores of Second World War pilots to return to their bases safely when their fuel was running low is helping to create a new breed of flying boats which could offer a highly efficient alternative to today's transocean transport aircraft and cargo ships. Known as "surface effect", the phenomenon occurs when an aircraft flies very low, at a height equal to one-half of its wing span or less. At such heights the aircraft creates a dynamic cushion of air that is trapped between the underside of its wings and the surface below. The closer the aircraft to the surface, the more effective the air cushion becomes. Flight within surface effect inhibits the downwash generated by wing lift, reducing induced drag by about 70 per cent. The reduction in downwash increases the overall lift-to-drag (L/D) ratio, which in turn reduces fuel consumption and permits the payload or the range to be increased.

Test craft have demonstrated that while a conventional aircraft at its normal flight altitude carries about 4kg (8.8lb) per hp of engine output, a craft designed to operate in surface effect carries up to 20kg (44lb), an improvement of 500 per cent. Research undertaken since the 1960s indicates that this new breed of flying boat — known as the Power-Augmented Ram Wing in Ground Effect Machine (PAR-WIG) in the West, and *ekranoplan* in the Soviet Union — will have a speed range of about zero (hovering) to 400kt (741km/hr; 461mph), be capable of non-stop flights of 2,600 to 4,340nm (4,828 to 8,047km; 3,000 to 5,000 miles), carry exceptionally heavy loads and be able to deliver these loads directly on to shorelines where necessary. They could prove to be the biggest single advance in ocean transport since the dawn of seafaring. All but the largest will have enough installed power to fly out of ground effect whenever necessary in order to clear shipping, shorelines, port installations, bends in rivers and fog banks.

The RFB X-114 experimental surface-effect craft, built in West Germany under a Federal Ministry of Defence contract.

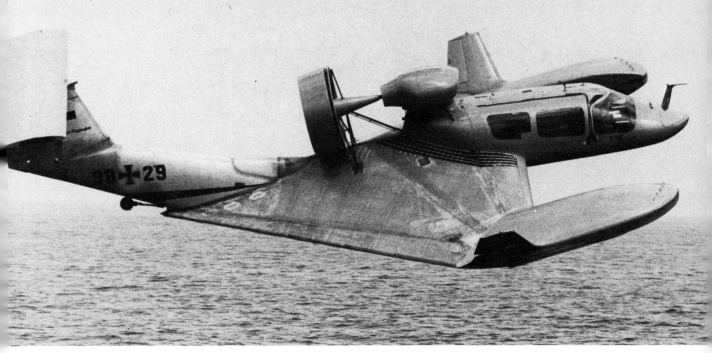

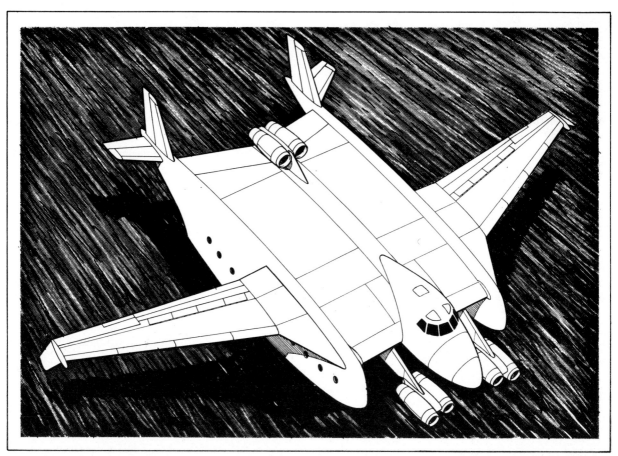

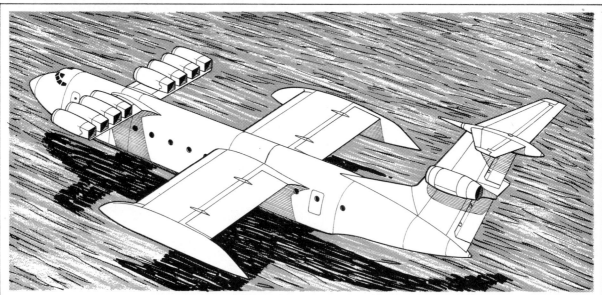

Top **Impression of a possible production version of a large twin-hulled ekranoplan designed in the Soviet Union by the late Robert Oros di Bartini.**

Above **The Soviet Union's Caspian Sea Monster.**

Efficiency, range and payload benefits

In full flight PAR-WIGs will manoeuvre in exactly the same way as aircraft, but out of surface effect their economic advantages are lost, since in order to maintain and gain height they have to operate at increased power. The fuel-consumption, range and payload benefits of flying in ground effect were recognised in the early days of commercial aviation. Lufthansa pilots operating flying boats over the South Atlantic in the 1930s frequently cruised only a few feet above the water, taking advantage of the layer of high-pressure air between their machines and the air-water interface. Employment of the technique not only extended the range of their aircraft by 50 per cent but also provided a remarkably smooth flight. Having trimmed their aircraft to fly on the air cushion and throttled back to about 25 per cent power, pilots found they were able to release their controls entirely, leaving the aircraft to fly themselves within the stability of the air cushion.

German flying-boat pilots were not alone in employing this technique. On one memorable occasion during the Second World War a badly damaged Short Sunderland was nursed back to base from far out in the Atlantic with only one of its four engines operating, a feat only made possible by the existence of surface effect.

Flying boats gradually waned in popularity after the war, despite the determined efforts of several air forces and airlines to retain them. Critics pointed to their inability to operate from points close to the world's main population centres, as few were (and few are today) located near waterways big enough to act as major flying-boat bases. Other disadvantages included the need for high installed thrust to counter the high drag present during take-off, and the need for particularly robust — and hence heavy — hull and wing structures to withstand wave impact on landing.

Since the new generation of flying boats will specialise in the carriage of freight or military equipment, and because of a more sophisticated approach to take-off and landing, these are no longer disadvantages. PAR-WIGs are viewed principally as vehicles capable of carrying perishable goods and other time-critical cargoes over long and medium distances more cheaply than aircraft and more quickly than ships. In the transport efficiency spectrum they fill a void in the middle speed range of 32-741km/hr (20-460mph), between the upper speed of conventional oceangoing cargo vessels and the lowest cruising speeds of jet aircraft. They could fly from port to port or base to base, but since the displacement draught of even a 5,000-tonne PAR-WIG would probably not exceed more than 3m (10ft), they would not be limited to operation from deepwater harbours or ports. Moreover, as mentioned earlier, the need of conventional flying boats for especially high installed thrust for take-off and heavy construction are obviated by using the PAR-WIG technique, which enables these craft to rise out of the water on

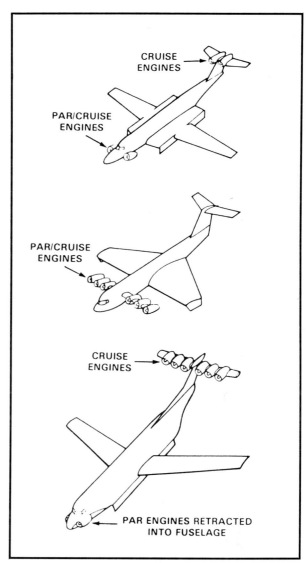

Three PAR-WIG studies examined by the US Marine Corps, which is considering this type of vehicle as a heavy-lift transport for its contribution to the Rapid Deployment Force. (C. Heber, DTNSRDC)

an air cushion before take-off and to set down at a low speed on an air cushion when landing in both rough and calm water. The same capability also permits land or shoreline landings.

Classical ram-wing configuration

In a typical aeroplane configuration a PAR-WIG incorporates a low-aspect-ratio mainplane with trailing-edge flaps and large endplates at its wingtips. With flaps extended the wing underside assumes a classical ram-wing configuration, similar to an upturned matchbox drawer with its front end removed. Ahead of and above the wing are propulsion jets, mounted either on a bridge or stub wing or recessed into the hull. Their exhaust deflectors are rotated downwards to direct their high-energy efflux into the open-fronted plenum framed by the wing underside, the endplates, flaps and

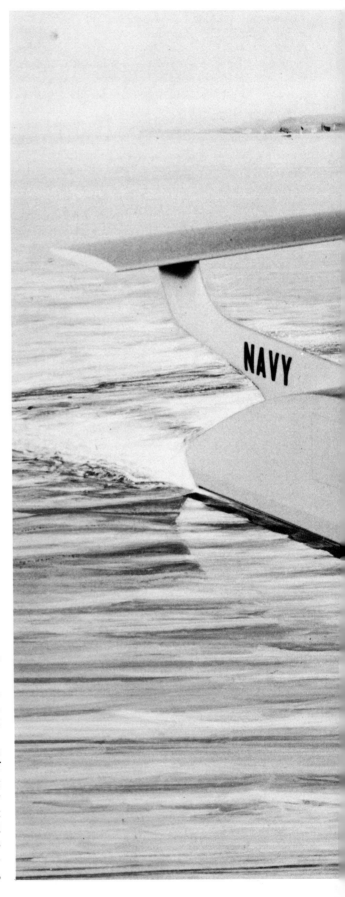

water surface beneath, and the craft is lifted bodily out of the water on a cushion of pressurised air.

As the machine rises on its cushion, it begins accelerating. As it approaches the onset of cushion hump drag, dynamic lift generated by the forward movement of the wings begins to supplement the static lift provided by the PAR cushion. Acceleration continues until the machine takes off and flies entirely supported by its dynamic surface-effect cushion. Once cruising speed has been reached, the thrust deflectors are rotated back to the horizontal position to align their efflux with the line of flight. Wing flaps are retracted and the craft is then trimmed to ride on the air cushion at a height which depends on the local sea state.

Within surface effect, the machine seeks its own stability height above rough water. Small test craft have completed many hours of operation in the Mediterranean and Baltic in quite high sea states. Designers have found that, provided the craft are soundly built and stable, impacts with the crests of above-average-height waves have no adverse effect on safety or performance.

Preliminary studies suggest that to avoid wave contact on a series of random flights over the North Atlantic the flying height would have to be no more than 1.8m (6ft) above mean water level at least 50 per cent of the time and no more than 3.6-4.5m (12-15ft) for 10 per cent of the time. These figures could however probably be improved upon very significantly with the aid of forecasts based on weather satellite observations and route planning to avoid storm centres. Sonic/electronic sensor systems would be employed to adjust flying height to changes in sea conditions.

Soviet developments

Billions of roubles have been poured into Soviet research and development programmes, which seem to have had the full backing of Krushchev, Brezhnev and Admiral of the Fleet of the Soviet Union S. G. Gorshkov. In his book *Sea Power of the State*, Gorshkov expresses his view that ekranoplans "will possess greater speed, use less fuel and have a greater range than conventional air-cushion vehicles, in addition to which they will be capable of clearing obstacles of great height."

Soviet aircraft design groups and naval architects have produced many thousands of analytical studies of ekranoplans covering every aspect of design from wing aerodynamics, flaps and controls to compressibility effects and endplates. There is no doubt that Soviet efforts will continue until the technology is perfected and machines enter service. Soviet military experts foresee wide employment of this type of vessel, particularly in the Soviet Navy, which, it has been suggested,

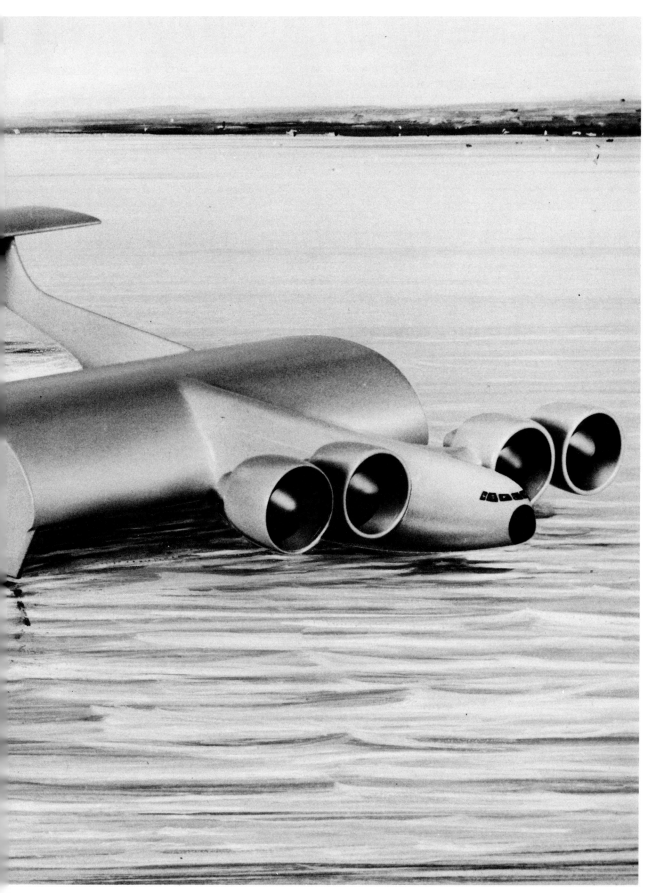

will find them invaluable in amphibious assault and resupply operations and for ASW patrol. Commercial variants will undoubtably one day be employed on express passenger and freight services on Soviet inland waterways and could ultimately appear on routes in the Baltic and Black Sea.

In the United States a programme to exploit the performance potential of surface effect was mounted under joint Navy and Army funding during the 1960s. Wind-tunnel experiments produced a wealth of data on the phenomenon. Unfortunately, the design studies that followed, while confirming the improvements in lift-to-drag ratios resulting from flying in surface effect, also indicated poor performance because the designs possessed the same take-off and landing disadvantages inherent in conventional flying boats. As a result, further investigations were suspended.

In the mid-1970s, however, during the preparation of the Advanced Naval Vehicle Concept Evaluation, wind tunnel, towing basin and free-flight model tests were conducted to check out the PAR technique, which Soviet designers had been applying to the "Caspian Sea Monster" and many other Soviet ekranoplan test craft since 1960. The tests showed that PAR-WIGs, with a jet efflux forward of the wing but deflected below the leading edge, could generate exceptionally high lift-to-thrust and lift-to-drag ratios up to 741km/hr (460mph), representing a significant advance on previous concepts.

Marine Corps enthusiasm

Currently one of the leading United States protagonists of PAR-WIG is the Marine Corps, which has been evaluating it as a quick-reaction vehicle for amphibious operations. Within US military circles the feeling is that if PAR-WIG is found to deliver its theoretical energy and investment advantages, and can also operate independently of runways, it will be the natural choice for a heavy military airlift vehicle for the 1990s.

PAR-WIG is also seen by the US military as a possible alternative to the C-5A heavy transport aircraft. Apart from its multi-terrain landing and take-off capability, it would also eliminate the threat of runway denial, an important consideration where aircraft like the C-5A are concerned. It would also make long-range round-trip flights a possibility, thus simplifying back-up problems.

The C-5A, one of the mainstays of a US Rapid Deployment Force, has a good maximum range fully loaded, but PAR-WIG can still score by offering greater range and payload capability, and at the same time provides far greater flexibility in the choice of landing areas and bases. A typical PAR-WIG configuration studied by the US Marine Corps would travel at 250-350kt (463-648km/hr; 288-403mph), have an all-up weight of 907,184kg (2,000,000lb) and be capable of travelling over 11,120km (6,900 miles) carrying a 340,194-385,550kg (750,000-850,000lb) payload. Employed in a Rapid Deployment Force role from bases on the US east and west coasts, these craft could reach almost any coastline in the world in three or four days.

The recent Falklands crisis highlights the enormous potential of such machines as high-speed transports and in other military roles. A squadron of PAR-WIGs could have reached the Falkland Islands in almost the same number of hours as it took days for the slow-moving conventional Task Force ships to complete the trip. The assault force and its vehicles, weapons and aircraft could have been on the spot long before the bulk of the invading force had established their defences. In the meantime, missile-equipped PAR-WIGs of the Royal Navy could have been patrolling the surrounding seas at speed, intercepting approaching troopships and hunting hostile submarines. UK defence planners should begin at once to examine their transport needs of the future. The PAR-WIG looks as if it could be the best and most cost-effective answer to many requirements.

If commercial users feel the same way, this new breed of skimmer is assured of a leading role in global transportation at the turn of the 21st century.

Jarrett's Jubilees

PHILIP JARRETT

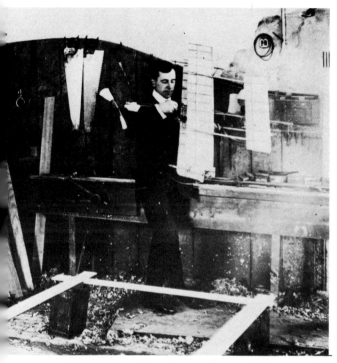

1907

While the Wright Brothers were bustling between the USA and Europe, busily bargaining with several nations (including their own) over the rights to build their developed biplane, European aeronautical activity was increasing. Following his success of 1906, Santos-Dumont had built and tested his No 15 tractor biplane, subsequently abandoned after a taxiing mishap on March 27. The Brazilian then set to work on a monoplane, the No 19.

Meanwhile, in England, the *Daily Mail* model aeroplane exhibition and competition, announced late the previous year, opened on April 6 in the Agricultural Hall, Islington, London. At the flying trials, held at the Alexandra Palace a week later, the rubber-powered models of A. V. Roe, then close to his 30th birthday, outflew all comers both indoors and outdoors. However, although the flights certainly qualified Roe for the £150 first prize by exceeding the specified 30.5m (100ft) minimum distance, the adjudicators decreed

A. V. Roe with his model aeroplane at home in 1906. *(P. Toobey)*

A. V. Roe I biplane at Brooklands in 1907. *(Flight)*

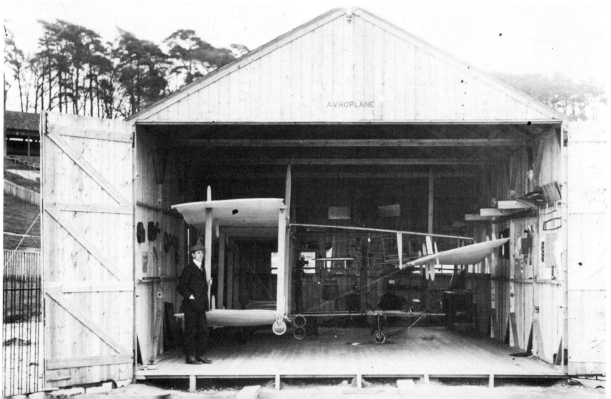

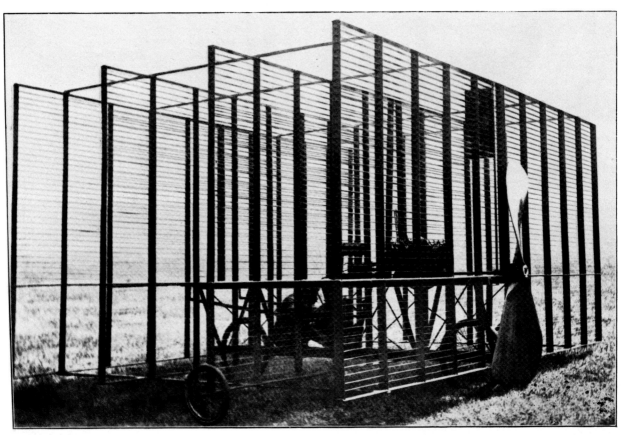

Phillips *Multiplane.*

that none of the models merited the full sum, and awarded Roe only the £75 second prize.

With this money, plus £500 won in cycle races, Roe began the construction of his first full-size machine, based upon the best of his models. Built in the stables behind his brother's doctor surgery in Putney, London, the aircraft was a primitive pusher biplane with a canard control surface, powered by a 6.7kW (9hp) JAP motorcycle engine driving a paddle-bladed propeller.

After its completion in September Roe moved the aircraft to the Brooklands motor racing track, where he planned to attempt to win a £2,500 prize offered by the owners for the first flight round the track before the end of the year. After much taxiing the biplane proved underpowered and only left the ground under tow, although its designer/pilot was able to familiarise himself with the controls.

A British aircraft of more eccentric design was the "venetian blind" *Multiplane* built by Horatio Phillips and tested at Streatham during the spring/summer period of the year. Comprising four frames each containing 50 thin "slat" wings, it was powered by a 15-16.4kW (20-22hp) engine which drove a 2.1m (7ft) diameter tractor propeller. Phillips reported its longitudinal stability to be "very satisfactory," but the machine apparently lacked any control surfaces. Several hops were made, including one of about 152m

(500ft), but the *Multiplane* progressed no further and influenced no one. Nonetheless, those hops, and some shorter ones in an earlier machine in 1903, are credited as being the first tentative powered flights in Britain.

Meanwhile, in a remote part of the British Isles, further interesting work was in progress. In 1906 Lt J. W. Dunne had been recruited by the Balloon Factory at Farnborough to develop his stable swept-wing tailless aircraft, and the first manned example, the D.I-A glider, was taken to the Atholl Hills in Scotland's Grampian Mountains in the early summer of 1907. After a few trials it crashed with Col Capper, Head of the Balloon School, aboard.

While being repaired the glider was converted into the D.I-B powered aircraft by the addition of a pair of 9kW (12hp) Buchet engines mounted co-axially and driving two propellers. However, after several unsuccessful attempts at flight the machine was badly damaged when it ran off its inclined timber track and pitched on to its nose. With winter fast approaching the team returned to Farnborough.

Denmark's J. C. Ellehammer tested his No III triplane on the outskirts of Copenhagen. Resembling his 1906 semi-biplane in most respects, the triplane was powered initially by a 15kW (20hp) three-cylinder engine and then by a five-cylinder radial that developed 26kW (35hp). Although Ellehammer claimed to have made about 200 hops in this aircraft before abandoning it, there was no proper means of achieving lateral con-

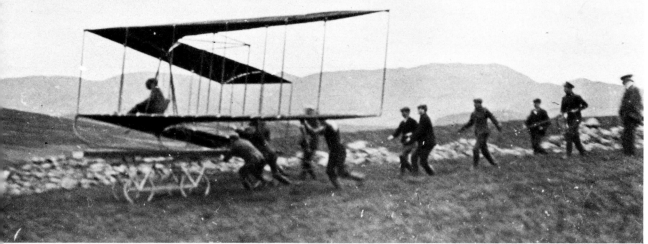

Testing a Dunne glider in the Atholl Hills in Scotland. *(Flight)*

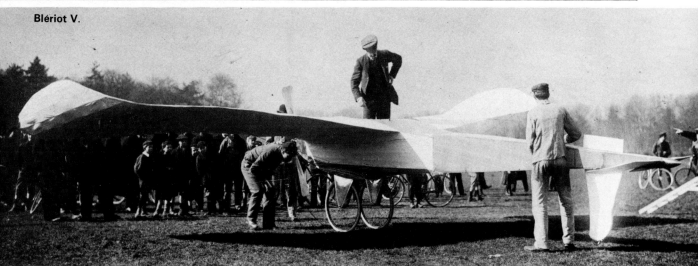

Blériot V.

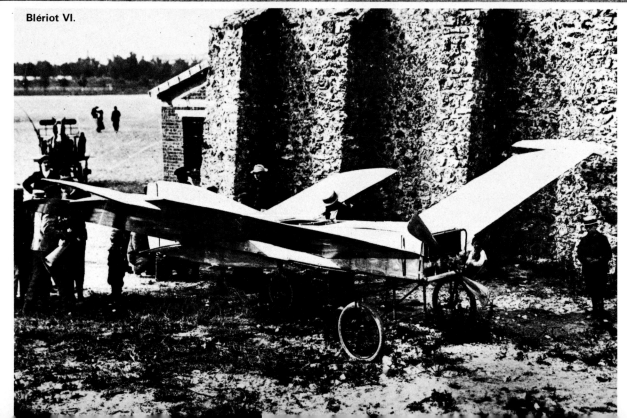

Blériot VI.

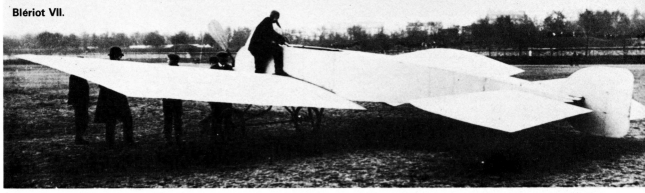

Blériot VII.

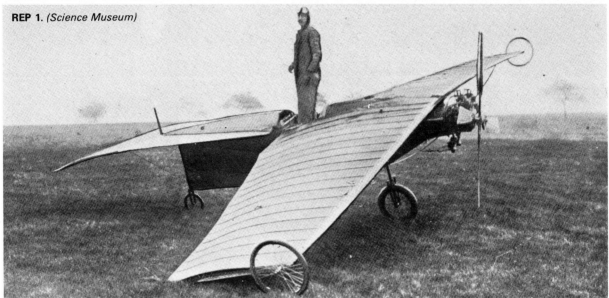

REP 1. (Science Museum)

trol, and the "rudder" was only a fabric cover over the rear landing wheel.

Much was also happening in France. Louis Blériot, working on the "build and test" principle, built three monoplanes of different configuration. First came the Blériot V, a canard aircraft with cambered wings that swept back at the tips. At the nose were an elevator and rudder, and primitive wing warping was also provided. An 18kW (24hp) Antoinette engine behind the pilot drove a two-bladed pusher propeller. The Blériot V was wrecked in April on its fourth take-off, never having bettered 6m (19ft) in the air.

The Blériot V was closely followed by the Langley-inspired Blériot VI tandem monoplane *Libellule* (Dragonfly), the first cantilever monoplane ever to be tested. This time the 18kW (24hp) Antoinette drove a tractor propeller, and wingtip elevons were fitted in addition to the large fin and rudder. During July and August 1907 it made 11 take-offs, six of which resulted in hop flights of more than 100m (328ft). Like all early aircraft, it was the subject of continuous modification, including the installation of a 37.3kW (50hp) Antoinette engine, which helped to push the weight up from 280kg (617lb) to 300kg (661lb). The Blériot VI made six further take-offs at Issy in September 1907,

four producing hops greater than 100m (328ft), the best covering 184m (600ft).

In the third machine, the No VII, Blériot turned to the classic tractor monoplane format. Powered by the 37.3kW (50hp) Antoinette driving a metal four-bladed propeller, the No VII spanned 11m (36ft) and featured mainplanes with marked dihedral, an enclosed fuselage, and an all-flying tail with rudder and large elevon surfaces. At Issy during November and December this aircraft made six flights, two of which each covered 500m (1,640ft). The No VII was to prove a trendsetter in monoplane design.

Another monoplane to appear in 1907 was the REP 1, bearing the initials of its creator, Robert Esnault-Pelterie, who had also produced its 22.4kW (30hp) seven-cylinder radial engine. This strange short-fuselaged machine had 9.6m (31ft 6in) span wings set at an anhedral angle and a fan-shaped tailplane and elevator, but lacked a rudder. The undercarriage comprised tandem mainwheels and auxiliary wingtip wheels. Promising hops were made during tests in November and December, 600m (1,968ft) being covered on November 16, but the monoplane was deficient in both longitudinal and directional stability.

Santos-Dumont's No 19 also made its debut late in

the year. A diminutive high-winged monoplane spanning only 5m (16ft 5in), it is now recognised as the progenitor of the ultra-light aeroplane. Its 15kW (20hp) Dutheil-Chalmers engine drove a two-blade metal tractor propeller, and it was controlled by means of a cruciform tail unit working in unison with a forward elevator surface. There was no means of lateral control other than by the pilot's rocking his body from side to side. The No 19's flying career was brief, consisting of only three take-offs, one each at Bagatelle, Issy and Buc, in November.

After testing a Chanute-type hang glider at Le Touquet in May 1907 the brothers Charles and Gabriel Voisin began to produce powered machines. First to take to the air was the Voisin-Delagrange No 1, built for Leon Delagrange and powered by a 37.3kW (50hp) Antoinette motor. It had a boxkite tail with twin rudders, and forward elevators, but lacked lateral control. After six take-offs at Bagatelle between March 16 and April 13, when it managed a 60m (197ft) hop, it was tested without success as a floatplane on Lake d'Enghien. After the land undercarriage was restored it made two take-offs at Issy on November 2 and 3 with

Delagrange in control, but was destroyed when it crashed following a 500m (1,640ft) hop on the second flight.

A Voisin was also ordered by the French-domiciled Englishman Henri Farman. Initially this machine closely resembled the Delagrange aircraft, but following tests in October a monoplane elevator replaced the biplane unit, and the wings were given dihedral. Later the tail unit was reduced in span. Between September 30 and November 23 this machine made some 20 take-offs at Issy, the most momentous flight covering a circular track of over 1,030m (3,379ft) in 1min 14sec on November 9. This was the first time that a non-Wright aeroplane had remained airborne for more than a minute, and had completed a circle. As the first officially recorded flight of 150m (492ft), it won Farman the Archdeacon Cup.

In America a 21-year-old named Glenn L. Martin was making tentative glides over Santa Ana, California, in a glider of his own design, and in neighbouring Canada Dr Alexander Graham Bell became chairman of the Aerial Experiment Association, formed on October 1. Financed by Mrs Bell, at whose suggestion

Santos-Dumont Demoiselle No 19.

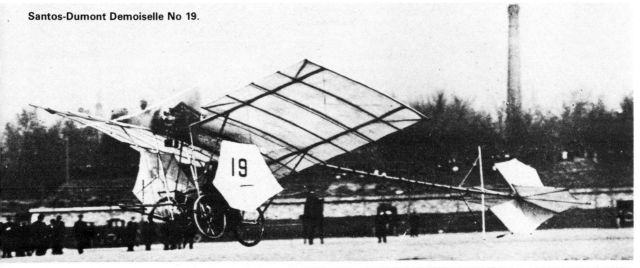

Voisin biplane flown by Henri Farman in November 1907.

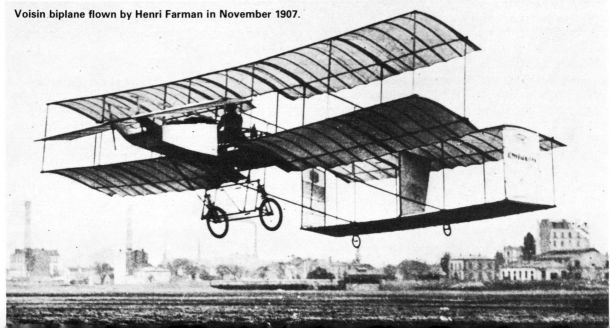

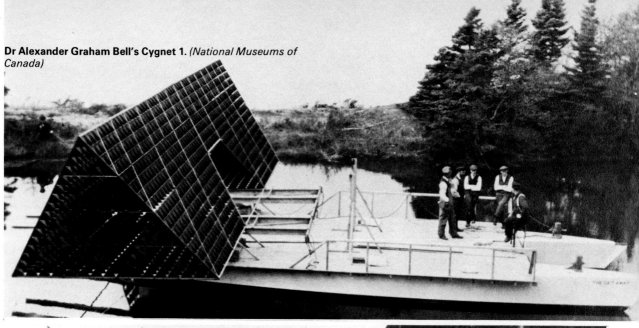

Dr Alexander Graham Bell's Cygnet 1. *(National Museums of Canada)*

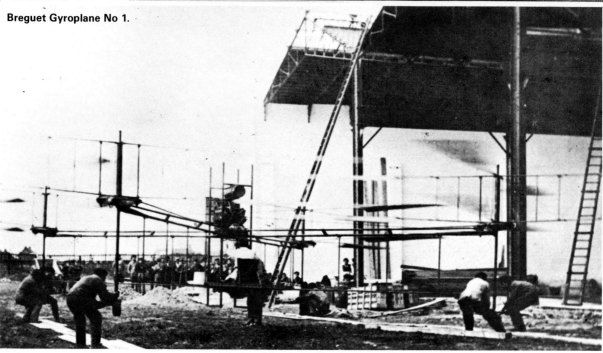

Breguet Gyroplane No 1.

it was formed, the AEA comprised Dr Bell, Glenn Curtiss, J. A. D. McCurdy, F. W. "Casey" Baldwin and Lt Thomas E. Selfridge, US Army. Their aim was to develop a powered aircraft. Work would take place at Bell's Beinn Bhreagh Laboratory and at Curtiss's Hammondsport site. The last months of 1907 were spent completing and testing Dr Bell's extraordinary tetrahedral-cell "aerodrome" kite, the *Cygnet* 1, of which the initial trial was made on December 3, under tow by a motor boat. A second trial, on December 6 with Lt Selfridge aboard the glider, ended in a ducking for Selfridge when the kite was inadvertently allowed to descend, towed at speed through the water and wrecked.

For heavier-than-air flight the year ended with the issue, by the US Army, of the first specification for

commercial tender of a military aeroplane. Dated December 23, it was drawn up by Chief Signal Officer Brig-Gen James Allen.

1907 was also a notable year for helicopters. On September 29 the Gyroplane No 1, built by Louis and Jacques Breguet in association with Prof Charles Richet, became the first machine to rise vertically from the ground by means of rotating wings, although it required four men to keep it steady. Only two months later, on November 13, another Frenchman, Paul Cornu, made the first piloted free flight in a rotorcraft, at Coquainvilliers, near Lisieux. The tandem-rotor machine weighed 190kg (419lb) with its 18kW (24hp) Antoinette engine. However, the flight lasted only about 20sec and the altitude reached was an unimpressive 0.30m (1ft). Problems with the structure, trans-

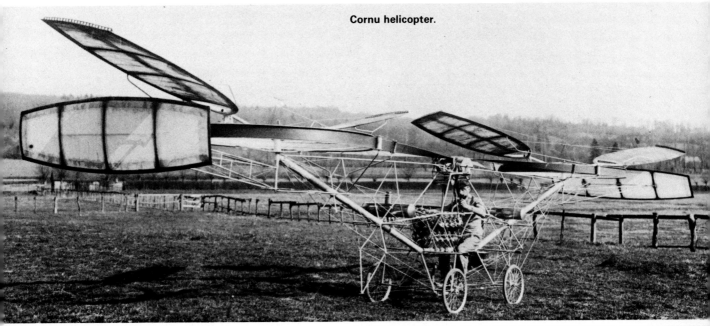

Cornu helicopter.

mission and controls, and a lack of finance, meant that this was the end of the experiments.

September 10 was the day when Britain's first military airship and its first practical airship, British Army Airship Dirigible No 1 *Nulli Secundus*, was launched "into the unstable ocean of the air" at Farnborough, Hampshire. A non-rigid airship, *Nulli Secundus* had two pusher propellers driven by a 37.3kW (50hp) Antoinette engine in the nacelle. Further test flights were made on September 30 and October 3. Then, on October 5, it was boldly decided to attempt a record trip to London. At 10.40 a.m., with Col Capper at the helm, the airship set off with the assistance of a gusty tailwind. *Nulli Secundus* reached St Paul's Cathedral at 12.20, turned around the famous dome and proceeded south, reaching Clapham Common at 1.10 p.m. The adverse wind had made the return flight much slower, and now forward speed was lost and a forced descent made in the grounds of the Crystal Palace at Sydenham at 2.07 p.m. Unfortunately the airship was torn loose from her temporary moorings by wind on October 10, and the envelope had to be slit open with a knife to prevent her breaking away completely. She would eventually re-emerge as *Nulli Secundus II*.

One notable ballooning event occurred in 1907. On October 12/13 the hydrogen balloon *Mammoth*, manned by the French aeronaut A. E. Gaudron and two others, made the first crossing of the North Sea by air. Ascending from the Crystal Palace, *Mammoth* covered a straight-line distance of some 1,160km (721 miles) before landing at Brackan on the shore of Lake Vänern, Sweden.

1932

Imperial Airways opened the year by extending its weekly England to Central Africa mail service from Kisumu to Cape Town. Inaugurated on January 20, the

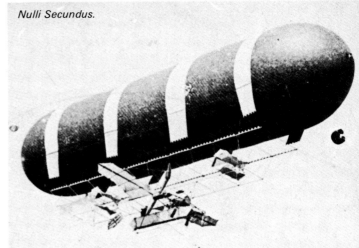

Nulli Secundus.

service carried its first mail from Croydon to Paris on Handley Page H.P.42W G-AAXF *Helena*. After transport by rail to Brindisi, the mail then went to Alexandria in a Short Scipio flying boat, where it was again transferred to another train for the journey to Cairo. There it was loaded aboard an Armstrong Whitworth Argosy, which flew it to Khartoum. The next leg, to Kisumu, was flown by a Short Calcutta flying boat. The final, newly established leg to Cape Town was flown by a de Havilland D.H.66 Hercules. Scheduled to complete the run in 11 days, the first mail to Cape Town reached its destination on February 2.

The first return mail flight, which started on January 27, did not go so smoothly. Leaving Cape Town in D.H.66 G-AARY *City of Karachi*, the mail was transferred to sister aircraft G-AAJH *City of Basra* at Johannesburg, but this machine hit an anthill and crashed at Salisbury on January 29. The mail was then loaded aboard a third D.H.66, G-EBMX *City of Delhi*. This

147

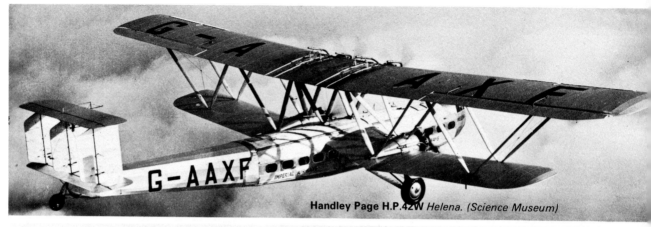

Handley Page H.P.42W *Helena. (Science Museum)*

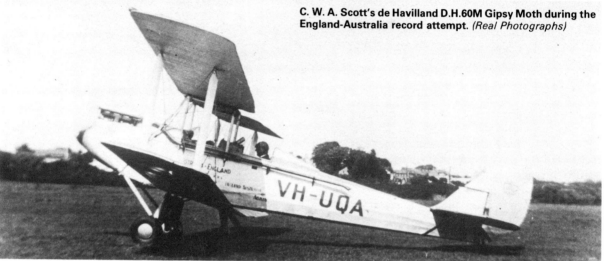

C. W. A. Scott's de Havilland D.H.60M Gipsy Moth during the England-Australia record attempt. *(Real Photographs)*

aircraft was forced down by a rainstorm on the same day near Broken Hill, and its cargo was not salvaged until February 4. Meanwhile, mail from Broken Hill and intermediate stops to Nairobi was carried in yet another D.H.66, G-EBMY *City of Baghdad*, which departed Broken Hill on February 2 and reached its destination the following day. The salvaged mail eventually reached London on the second weekly service, arriving on February 16.

On May 9 a significant step in air safety was marked by the accomplishment of the world's first solo flight under artificial blind-flying conditions. This occurred at Wright Field, with US Army Air Corps Capt Albert Hegenberger beneath the blind-flying hood of the specially modified and equipped Consolidated NY-2 trainer, originally supplied for the Guggenheim Fund's "Full Flight Laboratory" at Mitchel Field. Hegenberger remained under cover, without an accompanying check pilot, from take-off to touchdown.

Record-breaking flights abounded in 1932, just as they had in previous years, and only the most notable will be recorded here. At 10.45 a.m. on March 24 James A. Mollison, who had claimed the Australia-to-England record in 1931, took off from Lympne, Kent, in long-range de Havilland Puss Moth G-ABKG, powered by an 89kW (120hp) Gipsy III engine, and set course to follow the West Coast route to Cape Town, South Africa. Mollison touched down on the beach at Milnerton, only three miles from his intended destination, at 8.35 p.m. on March 28. The Puss Moth was damaged and he could fly no further, but he had made the 10,227km (6,355-mile) flight in four days 17hr 30min, knocking some 13hr off the record set by Peggy Salaman and A. Gordon Store in 1931.

A month later, on April 19, C. W. A. Scott set out from Lympne at 5.05 a.m. in de Havilland D.H.60M Gipsy Moth VH-UQA in an attempt to regain the England-Australia record taken from him by C. A. Butler. He completed the journey at 10.22 a.m. on April 28, having covered the distance in eight days, 20hr 47min to clip 5hr 42min off the previous best. The North Atlantic was flown on several occasions, the first crossing of the year going to the credit of Mrs G. P. Putnam (previously and better known as Amelia Earhart), who left New Jersey, USA, in her 313kW (420hp) Pratt & Whitney Wasp-powered Lockheed Vega on May 19. Next day, two hours after her arrival at Harbour Grace, Newfoundland, she took off to make the first coast-to-coast solo Atlantic crossing by a woman. Despite deteriorating weather and technical problems—a leaky fuel gauge, faulty altimeter and broken exhaust manifold—the coast of Donegal, Ireland, was crossed at 11.45 a.m. local time on May 21. At 13hr 15min the crossing was the fastest to date. Mrs Putnam then "Bradshawed" along a railway line to Londonderry, landed on a farm at Culmore, and later flew on to London.

On the same day that Mrs Putnam set off, D-1929, the massive Dornier Do X flying boat powered by no fewer than 12 447kW (600hp) Curtiss Conqueror 12-cylinder water-cooled engines mounted in tandem pairs above its 48m (157ft 6in) span wing, lifted off from New York to return to Europe as part of a continuing "long distance test flight" that had started at Altenrhein on November 5, 1930. After a stopover at St John's, Newfoundland, on May 21, the aircraft flew on to the Azores, which were reached in darkness and fog. Vigo on the Spanish coast was reached the next day, and on May 23 the flying boat visited Southamp-

ton, England, before flying home to Germany. Her commander, Capt Christiansen, put her down on the Miggelsee in Berlin on May 24, thereby ending a truly epic voyage.

While Amy Johnson was in Australia in 1930 she had met Jim Mollison, and in London on July 29, 1932, the two record-breakers were married. Shortly afterwards, on August 18, Jim Mollison was off yet again, this time on the first New York return-flight attempt. His mount was de Havilland D.H.80A Puss Moth G-ABXY *The Heart's Content*, powered by the reliable and economical Gipsy III engine. The aircraft was virtually standard, but the wheel and airbrakes had been removed, controls and instruments moved aft to make room for a 284lit (75 US gal) fuel tank in the forward cabin area, and a 178lit (47 US gal) tank positioned behind the seat. The two standard 76lit (20 US gal) wing tanks were retained. Taking off from the beach at Portmarnock Strand, near Dublin, at 11.35 a.m., Jim Mollison

Jim Mollison's Puss Moth *The Heart's Content. (Flight)*

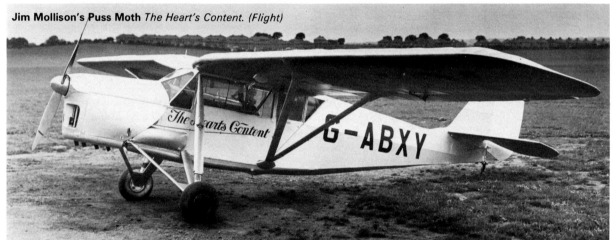

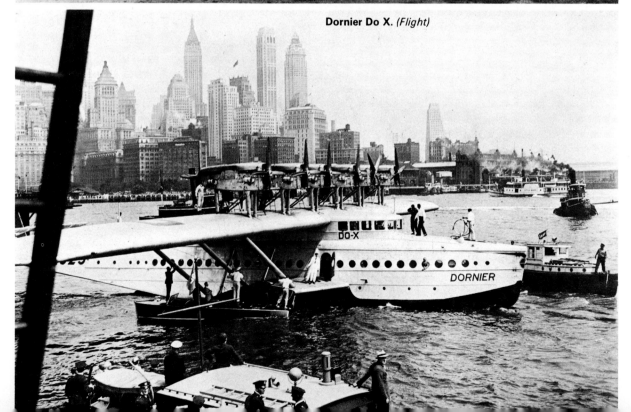

Dornier Do X. *(Flight)*

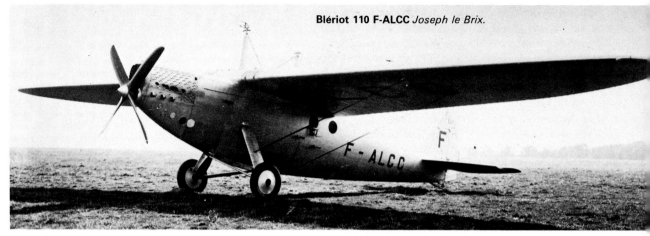

Blériot 110 F-ALCC *Joseph le Brix.*

headed steadily west and covered 4,184km (2,600 miles) in 22½hr, making landfall at Harbour Grace, Newfoundland. Just 24hr after take-off he was circling over Halifax, Nova Scotia, achieving an average speed for the trip of 161km/hr (100mph). Heading south for New York, Mollison became lost in mist and cloud and finally landed at Pennfield Ridge, New Brunswick, at 11.45 a.m. local time on August 19. The last 241km (150 miles) had taken 6hr, and only 45.5lit (10 US gal) of fuel remained.

Although his Puss Moth was in immaculate condition, Mollison was the worse for wear. Following medical advice, he abandoned his planned return flight and sailed home. Nonetheless, he had made the first east-west solo Atlantic crossing, the first lightplane crossing of the North Atlantic, and the longest non-stop flight to date by a light aircraft.

Not to be outdone by her husband, Amy Mollison set out to attack the South Africa-England record that he had established in March. At 6.37 a.m. on November 14 she took off from Lympne in another D.H.80A Puss Moth, G-ACAB *Desert Cloud*, powered by one of the first examples of the new 97kW (130hp) Gipsy Major engine. She landed at Cape Town at 3.31 p.m. on November 18, having covered 9,978km (6,200 miles), to set a new record time of four days 6hr 54min, almost 10½hr inside her husband's time. Amy then left Cape Town at 7 a.m. on December 11, her sights set on claiming the record for the return trip. In this she succeeded, touching down at Croydon at 12.45 p.m. on December 18 and establishing a new record time of seven days 7hr 5min.

Another type of distance record, that for distance in a closed circuit without refuelling, was won for France by Lucien Bossoutrot and Maurice Rossi during March 23-26, 1932. Flying the purpose-built 26.5m (87ft) span Blériot 110 high-wing monoplane F-ALCC *Joseph le Brix*, powered by a 447kW (600hp) Hispano-Suiza 12-cylinder Vee engine, they made a flight of 10,601.480km (6,587.442 miles) at Oran in Algeria.

On August 13, 1932, a startling new racing mono-plane took to the air for the first time at Springfield, Massachussets, in the USA. The Gee Bee R-1 Super Sportster, produced by Grenville Brothers Aircraft, was in essence a flying engine. A 544kW (730hp) Pratt & Whitney Wasp T3D1 nine-cylinder radial engine was mounted at the front of a barrel-like fuselage, and the pilot was positioned right in the tail in an enclosed cockpit which was faired directly into the minimal fin and deep rudder.

Both the R-1 and its sister, R-2 NR2101, participated in the US National Air Races at Cleveland, Ohio, that August/September. On September 3, 1932, James Doolittle flew the R-1 over the regulation FAI 3km course to achieve a new world landplane record speed of 476.828km/hr (296.287mph). Two days later Doolittle capped his achievement by winning the Thompson Trophy Race in the R-1, averaging 406.659km/hr (252.686mph) around ten laps of the 16km (10-mile) course.

1932 was quite a year for altitude records. On August 18/19 Auguste Piccard, a Swiss professor of physics at Brussels Technical College, made an attempt to beat his own world absolute altitude record of 15,781m (51,775ft) in a stratosphere balloon and gondola of his own design. Ascending from Dubendorf Airport, Zurich, in company with Dr Max Cosyns, Piccard took sufficient oxygen for 32hr. At 5 p.m. on the 19th the balloon landed near Lake Garda in Italy, having established a new record of 16,700m (54,789ft).

The altitude record for conventional aeroplanes was claimed by Britain on September 16. The pilot was Capt Cyril F. Uwins, chief test pilot of the Bristol Aeroplane Company, and his mount was Vickers Vespa VII G-ABIL. The 15.2m (50ft) span aircraft was selected for the record attempt because it was the only machine available with the necessary wing area (53.51m²; 576ft²) and high-lift capability at high altitudes.

Fitted with a Bristol Pegasus "S" supercharged engine driving a large-diameter two-blade propeller, G-ABIL reached 13,404m (43,976ft). This beat the then current American record by more than 244m

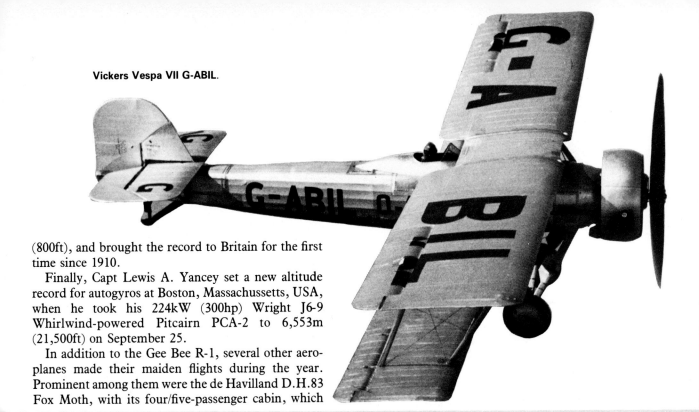

Vickers Vespa VII G-ABIL.

(800ft), and brought the record to Britain for the first time since 1910.

Finally, Capt Lewis A. Yancey set a new altitude record for autogyros at Boston, Massachussetts, USA, when he took his 224kW (300hp) Wright J6-9 Whirlwind-powered Pitcairn PCA-2 to 6,553m (21,500ft) on September 25.

In addition to the Gee Bee R-1, several other aeroplanes made their maiden flights during the year. Prominent among them were the de Havilland D.H.83 Fox Moth, with its four/five-passenger cabin, which

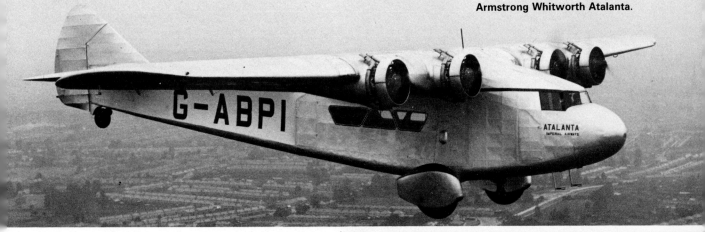

Armstrong Whitworth Atalanta.

first flew on January 29; Gloster's enormous TC-33 four-engined bomber-transport biplane (February 23); the Boeing XP-936, prototype of the celebrated P-26 "peashooter" monoplane fighter (March 20); the Airspeed Ferry airliner (April 5); Junkers Ju 52/3m (April); the four-seat ST-4, first product of the newly formed General Aircraft Company (May); Armstrong Whitworth's AW XV Atalanta four-engined high-wing monoplane airliner for Imperial Airways (June 6), which went into service on September 26; the Short Sarafand large six-engined biplane flying boat (June 30); the Handley Page H.P.46 shipborne torpedo bomber (October 25); and, finally, the de Havilland D.H.84 Dragon twin-engined biplane short-haul airliner, designed and built at the request of Edward Hillman, founder of Hillman's Airways (November 24). The first Dragon was delivered to the airline at Maylands Aerodrome, Romford, Essex, on December 20.

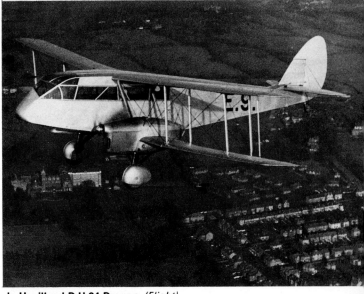

de Havilland D.H.84 Dragon. (Flight)

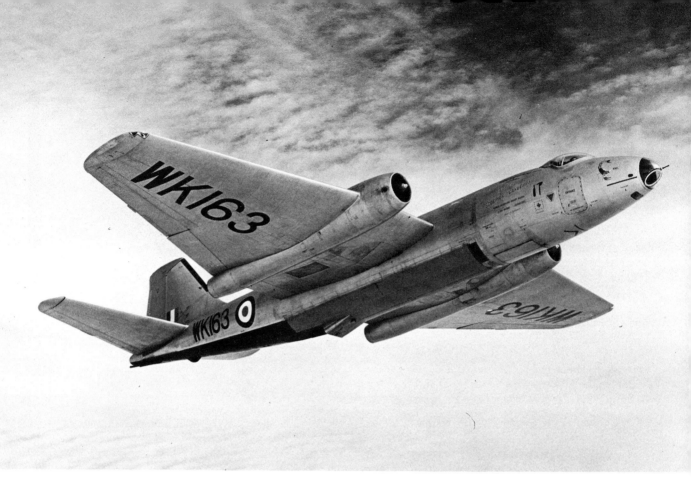

English Electric Canberra B.2 WK163. *(Flight)*

1957

In 1957 there were some curious parallels with 1932 as far as records were concerned. A world speed record was broken by America, the altitude record was broken by Britain, and a new balloon altitude record was established.

The balloon record was set on August 19/20 when Maj David G. Simons, a US Air Force medical officer, reached 30,942m (101,516ft) in the AF-WRI-I 84,950m³ (3,000,000ft³) balloon. With the intention of gathering scientific data on the stratosphere, Simons ascended from Crosby, Minnesota, and landed the following day at Frederick, South Dakota. It was the first ratified altitude record for a manned balloon to exceed 30,480m (100,000ft).

Compared with this the 21,430m (70,308ft) reached by D. Napier & Sons' testbed English Electric Canberra seems low, but for a manned jet bomber it was no mean achievement. However, a great deal of assistance was provided by a Napier Double Scorpion rocket motor installed in the bomb bay. The Napier aircraft, Canberra B.2 WK163, had passed 20,726m (68,000ft) between eight and twelve times during trials, and as it was clear that there was more than enough power in the Double Scorpion pack to do the job, it was decided to make the attempt.

On August 28 Michael Randrup, Napier's chief test pilot, and deputy chief engineer Walter Shirley took off from Luton, Bedfordshire, headed south-west and then turned eastwards over the Channel to the south of the Isle of Wight. At 13,411m (44,000ft) Randrup throttled the Canberra's two Rolls-Royce Avon turbojets to cruising r.p.m., switched on both barrels of the Scorpion, and the aircraft climbed at "a very steep angle" to 21,336m (70,000ft), where the rockets were switched off. The main function of the Avons at this time was simply to maintain pressurisation and to keep generators and other services going.

Very accurate flying was required, because at extreme altitudes an aeroplane's aerodynamic stalling speed approaches its limiting Mach number. In the case of the Canberra, although it had a relatively low stalling speed, its limiting Mach number was equally low by the standards of the time, and Randrup had to keep the bomber within a 28km/hr (17.5mph) safe speed range just above the 185km/hr (115mph) mark, with very poor external visual references and with the Scorpions pushing the machine up at a pronounced angle.

The world absolute speed record, previously held by Britain's Peter Twiss and the Fairey F.D.2 at 1,821.39km/hr (1,132mph), was pushed up to 1,943.5km/hr (1,207.633mph) on December 12, 1957. The man who claimed it was Maj Adrian E. Drew of the USAF, and his mount was McDonnell F-101A Voodoo single-seat fighter 32426. The flight was made at Edwards Air Force Base, the experimental centre on Muroc Dry Lake. At the time the Voodoo, powered by two Pratt & Whitney J57-P-13 turbojets, was only the third twin-engined aircraft to take the record since its inception.

Another record claimed by the USA in 1957 was that for distance in a straight line. This fell to a USAF Boeing KC-135A piloted by Gen Curtis E. LeMay and crew. The aircraft took off from Westover on November 12 and landed at Buenos Aires, Argentina, having covered (10.175.670km (6,322.856 miles).

Nearly a month earlier, on October 16, John Cunningham, piloting de Havilland Comet 3 G-ANLO, had established a new point-to-point speed record for the flight from Hatfield, Hertfordshire, to Khartoum, covering the 4,931km (3,064 miles) in 5hr 51min 14.8sec, an average speed of 842.2km/hr (523.4mph). He capped this on October 23-24 by flying the same aircraft from London to Johannesburg in 12hr 59min 7.3sec, averaging 697.8km/hr (433.6mph) for another point-to-point record in its class.

One further point-to-point record is worthy of mention. On May 25 Canberra PR.7 WT528 *Aries V* left Tokyo, Japan, at 11 p.m. and reached West Malling, Kent, 12,892km (8,011 miles) distant, in 17hr 42min 2.4sec. A new Tokyo-London record was credited to its crew, pilots Wg Cdr W. Hay and Flt Lt J. L. Dennis, and navigator Sqn Ldr B. Hamilton.

If 1957 was notable for one particular aircraft type, it should be remembered as the year of the Britannia. On February 1 BOAC put the world's first long-range turboprop-powered transport aircraft into scheduled service. The route on which these elegant Bristol Proteus-engined airliners were inaugurated was the thrice-weekly operation from London to Rome, Khartoum, Nairobi, Salisbury and Johannesburg on a 22hr 50min schedule. The honour of making the first run fell to G-ANBI, which reached Johannesburg on February 2. The return flight commenced the following day.

On June 29 the prototype of a long-range Britannia variant, the Series 310, registered G-AOVA, made the first ever non-stop airliner flight from London to the Pacific coast of Canada, when, on a proving flight, it covered the 8,207km (5,100 miles) to Vancouver in 14hr 40min. Still later in the year, on December 19, the production version of the 310, designated Series 312, inaugurated the first turbine-powered direct London-New York service. Pilot for the run was Capt A. Meagher, and his aircraft, G-AOVC, also flew the first eastbound flight two days later.

Maj Adrian E. Drew with his McDonnell F-101A Voodoo record-breaking fighter. *(Associated Press)*

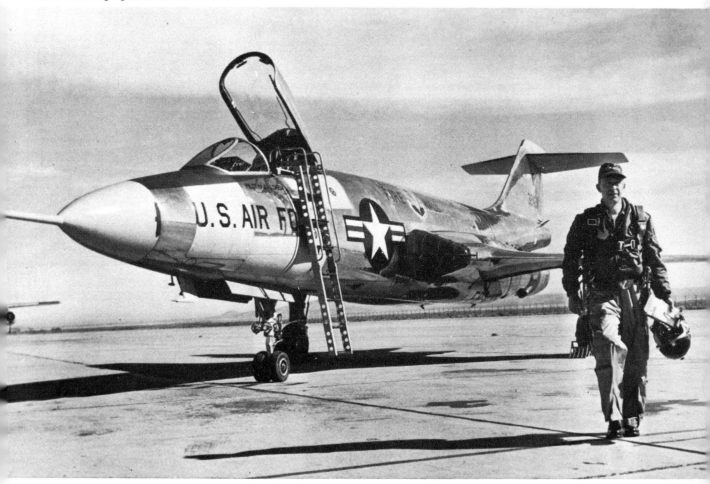

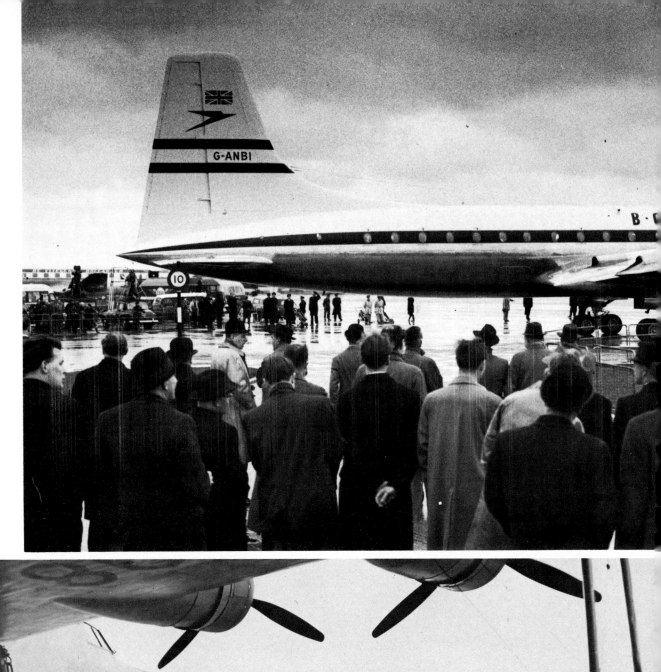

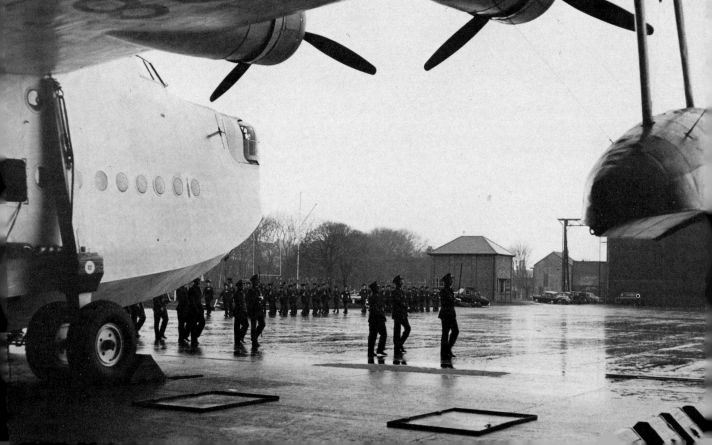

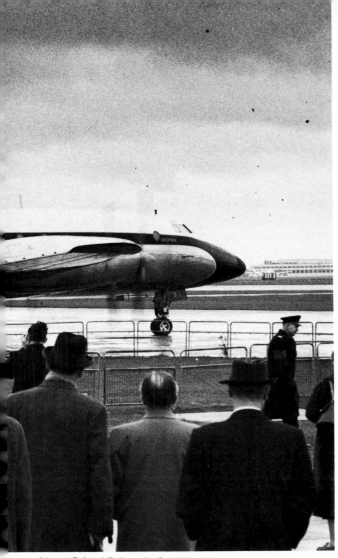

On the same day that the Britannia entered service, a ceremony was held in miserable weather at Pembroke Dock to pay a farewell tribute to one of the Royal Air Force's great aircraft. The Short Sunderland flying boat had first flown on October 16, 1937, and had entered RAF service with 230 Sqn the following year. Twenty years later that same squadron, in company with No 201, was disbanded, marking the demise of the military flying boat in Britain. The Sunderland had spent 17 years on first-line duties with Coastal Command, a longer period in such duties in its original designed role than any other RAF aircraft. In fact it was only an "official" farewell, for a few Sunderlands were to remain in service in the Far East with the combined 205/209 Sqn at Seletar before being replaced by Shackletons from the beginning of 1958.

While the RAF said goodbye to an old friend, the Royal Navy was greeting a new one. On March 20 the first production de Havilland Sea Vixen FAW.1 twin-boom, twin-engined all-weather fighter, XJ474, made its maiden flight at Christchurch powered by a pair of 44.5kN (10,000lb st) Rolls-Royce Avon turbojets. After trials at Boscombe Down, RAE Bedford, and afloat in HMS *Ark Royal* and HMS *Centaur* (this machine and XJ475), Y Flight of No 700 Sqn Service Trials Unit began a working-up programme in November 1957. Using early production Sea Vixens, this programme included three weeks in HMS *Victorious*.

Following its RAF debut with No 230 Operational Conversion Unit in 1956, Avro's delta-winged Type 698 medium bomber, better known as the Vulcan, entered service with 83 Sqn in July 1957 at Waddington, Lincolnshire, as part of Bomber Command's deterrent force. Powered by four Bristol Olympus tur-

Above **Bristol Britannia G-ANBI.** *(Flight)*

Left **Goodbye to the Sunderland.** *(Flight)*

Below **de Havilland Sea Vixen FAW.1 XJ474.** *(de Havilland)*

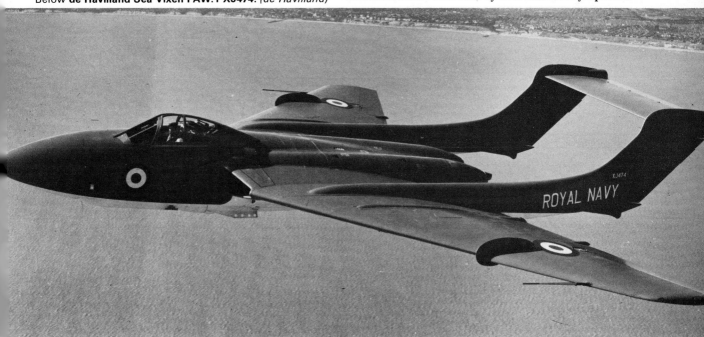

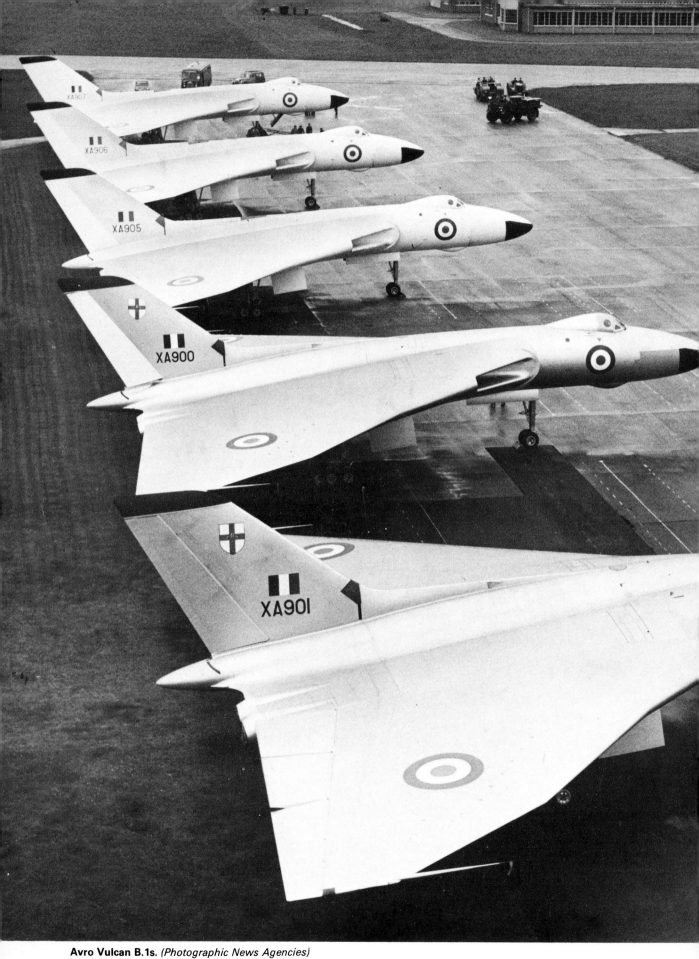

Avro Vulcan B.1s. *(Photographic News Agencies)*

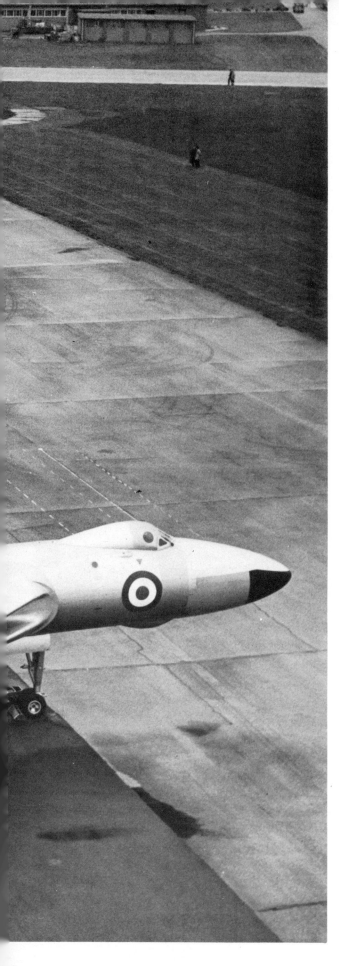

bojets, the Vulcan was the embodiment of designer Roy Chadwick's unconventional solution to the problem of combining high top speed with relatively low landing speed, while also meeting a demanding specification.

The pilots found their new mount "docile and gentlemanly" in its handling characteristics, and, as if to prove the point, aircrew from No 83 Sqn gained four awards in Bomber Command's 1957 Bombing and Navigation Competition. In its B.2 form the Vulcan has remained in service to the present day, being reprieved from the scrap merchant's torch at the eleventh hour by the Falklands crisis.

Meanwhile, A. V. Roe in Canada had been working on a delta of its own. On October 4 at the company's Malton, Ontario, plant the country's first supersonic aircraft, the CF-105 Arrow all-weather fighter, was rolled off the final assembly line. A massive 15.2m (50ft) span aircraft with 60° of sweepback on its high-set wing, it originated from a 1952 RCAF requirement. The first prototype (25201) was fitted with a pair of 102.3kN (23,000lb st) Pratt & Whitney J75 jet engines, but two 124.6kN (28,000lb st) Orenda Iroquois units were intended for production aircraft. Although it was anticipated that the new fighter would fly before the end of the year, it was not until well into 1958 that it finally left the ground.

First flights in 1957 were numerous, and the variety amazing. It included the tandem two-seat trainer variant of Lockheed's F-104 Starfighter, the F-104B, which took to the air in January, and, over in France, the bizarre Hurel-Dubois H.D.34 high-aspect ratio-wing aircraft for the Institut Géographique Nationale, which flew on February 26. Just over a month later, on March 28, Canadair's CL-28 Argus piston-engined maritime patrol aircraft, forerunner of the CL-44, flew for the first time. Three days later the Breguet 1100-01 fighter prototype exceeded Mach 1 in a shallow dive on its maiden flight. Another machine fledged on the same day was the Miles HDM 105, a British-built high-aspect-ratio twin displaying strong Hurel-Dubois influence.

Britain's English Electric P.1B, which formed the basis of the standard production Lightning single-seat fighter, took to the air on April 5, and another Miles prototype, the twin-finned M.100 Student side-by-side jet trainer, was flown by George Miles at Shoreham on May 15. The next day, at the Aeroplane and Armament Experimental Establishment, Boscombe Down, Wiltshire, test pilot John Booth took off in the Saunders-Roe SR-53, an experimental mixed-power interceptor powered by an Armstrong Siddeley Viper turbojet and a de Havilland Spectre rocket motor. Their combined power allowed it to reach 15,240m (50,000ft) in 2.2min. The next day, May 17, the Westland Wessex helicopter flew. The prototype was an imported Sikorsky S-58 airframe modified to accommodate the

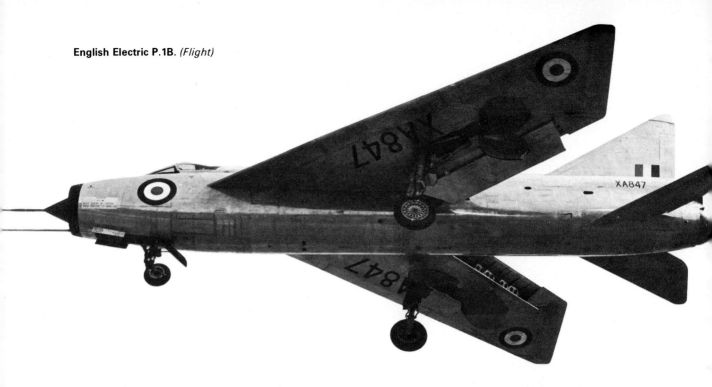

English Electric P.1B. *(Flight)*

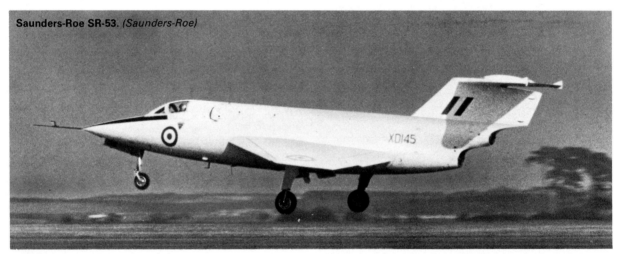

Saunders-Roe SR-53. *(Saunders-Roe)*

Napier Gazelle gas turbine in place of the original Wright R-8120-84 piston engine.

At Southend on July 9 a new medium-range 28-passenger airliner, the Rolls-Royce Dart-powered Aviation Traders ATL 90 Accountant, left the ground. It was doomed to remain a one-off type, but the man behind it, one Freddie Laker, had greater things ahead of him. In France the Breguet BR.1001 Taon lightweight ground-attack fighter, designed to meet a Nato specification and powered by a Bristol Olympus turbojet, flew for the first time on July 26. In the USA on September 4, only 241 days after its development had been authorised, Lockheed's CL-329 Jetstar light utility jet transport and crew readiness trainer for the USAF took to the skies. Although the prototype (N329J) had a pair of Orpheus engines in its rear-fuselage nacelles, subsequent examples were fitted with four General Electric J85 units.

The USSR's Tu-114 Rossiya (Russia) commercial transport first flew on October 3. Combining the wings, tail unit, undercarriage and four Kuznetsov 11,033kW (14,795ehp) NK-12M turboprops of the Tu-20 bomber with a new and enlarged fuselage, the Tu-114 could carry up to 220 passengers. After protracted trials, during which a number of international records were set in its class, the 51m (167ft) span airliner—the world's largest until the Boeing 747 appeared—was introduced on Aeroflot's non-stop Moscow-Khabarovsk service on April 24, 1961. Another Russian giant ends the list. On October 30 the largest helicopter in the world, Mikhail Mil's Mi-6, made its maiden flight. With a length of 33.18m (108ft 10½in) and a rotor diameter of 35m (114ft 10in), it was powered by two 3,505kW (4,700shp) Soloviev D-25 turboshafts.

In the promising field of vertical take-off and landing

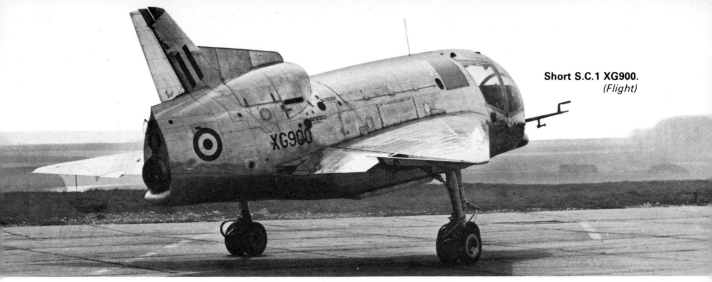

Short S.C.1 XG900.
(Flight)

(Vtol) 1957 was a vintage year. On April 2 at Boscombe Down a small, tubby-fuselaged delta-wing aeroplane made a conventional take-off and landing. However, the aircraft, Short S.C.1 XG900, was far from conventional. Although only the RB.108 propulsion unit was fitted at this time, the fuselage had provision for four vertically mounted RB.108s positioned around the centre of gravity and with their effluxes directed downwards to provide vertical lift. But Vtol was a new game, and Short's test pilot, Tom Brooke-Smith, had to gain experience by undertaking a helicopter conversion course and mastering the Rolls-Royce Thrust Measuring Rig, the famous "Flying Bedstead". The first hoving flight and first transition were still many months away.

Only a few days later, in the USA, another small delta-winged aircraft did make a complete transition cycle successfully. On April 11 the USAF's Ryan X-13 Vertijet rose up nose-first on the power of its Rolls-Royce Avon turbojet, curved over into horizontal flight and then settled back into a vertical landing. As the USA's first jet-powered Vtol aircraft, it had previously made the world's first jet Vtol transition—from conventional take-off and flight to hover — on November 28, 1956. Regrettably, the success on April 11 also marked the beginning of the end of USAF interest, and the work was soon discontinued.

Despite the setbacks that bedevilled Vtol research, there was no shortage of contenders. On April 21 the US Army's Vertol 76 was completed. Heralded as the world's first tilt-wing aircraft, the Vertol 76 had taken just 50 weeks to design and build. A single 597kW (800hp) Avco Lycoming T53 engine mounted on top of the rear fuselage drove the two contra-rotating propellers at the tips of the wings, which could be rotated through 90° from the vertical take-off to level-flight positions. Additional control in the hover was provided by two ducted fans in the base of the fin. The Vertol 76 made its first free flight on August 13 after a series of taxiing tests and tethered hovering flights, but its first transition had to wait until July 1958, and little resulted from the project.

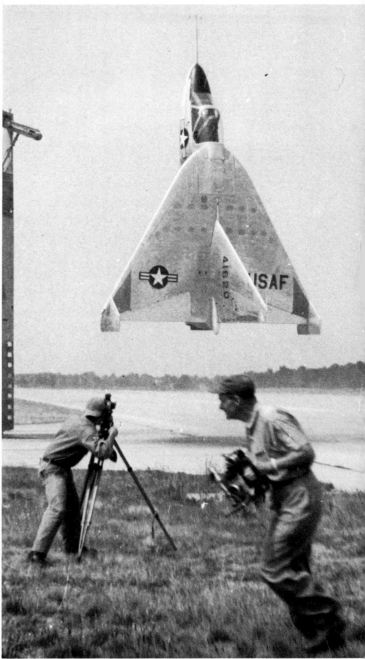

Ryan X-13 Vertijet. (Ryan)

159

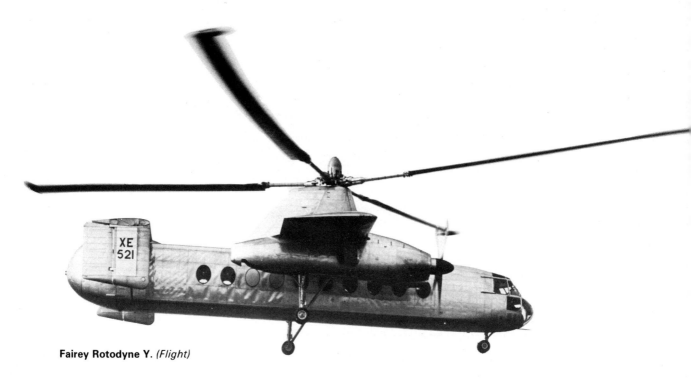

Fairey Rotodyne Y. *(Flight)*

Another dead-end Vtol type to appear in the USA during 1957 was Bell's X-14 for the USAF, which made its first hovering flight on February 19. It was powered by a pair of 7.8kN (1,750lb) thrust Armstrong Siddeley ASV.8 Viper turbojets mounted horizontally in the forward fuselage, their jetstream being deflected through diverters or vanes in the underfuselage. Control in the hover was effected by air jets in the wingtips and tail.

The last of the Vtol types to fly in 1957 was also the most ambitious and the most fully developed. The Fairey Aviation Company's Rotodyne Y 40-passenger Vtol transport aircraft was conceived in the late 1940s. British European Airways confirmed the need for a short/medium-haul convertiplane in 1951, and the completed aircraft (XE521) made its first flight at White Waltham, Berkshire, on November 6, 1957, piloted by W. R. Gellatly and J. G. P. Morton. The Rotodyne had a boxy fuselage from which sprouted 14.17m (46ft 6in) stub wings. Mounted on these were two 2,088kW (2,800shp) Napier Eland turboprops which turned a pair of four-blade propellers and also drove auxiliary compressors to power the pressure jets in the tips of a massive 27.4m (90ft) diameter four-blade rotor. A planned production version, the 70-passenger Rotodyne Z, was to be powered by Rolls-Royce Tynes.

Watching the Rotodyne take-off was a stirring—and deafening—experience. Following a vertical take-off the machine became an autogyro, the rotor autorotating while the turboprops provided forward thrust and the wings provided much of the lift. The first transition to and from autogyro mode was made on April 10, 1958, and the Rotodyne flew on for four years, making many public appearances until the cancellation of the programme in February 1962.